CONFESSIONS
of an
ESTROGEN
EVANGELIST

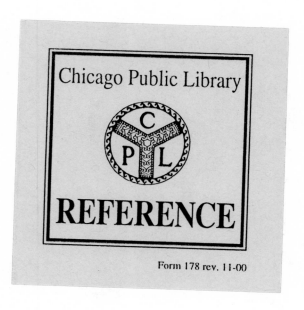

CONFESSIONS
of an
ESTROGEN
EVANGELIST

• • •

Setting the Record Straight on
Estrogen Replacement Therapy

• • •

JOYCE A. KAKKIS, M.D.,
and DAVID PAUL GREEN

To Peter
My soul mate and love
of my life, for his
unwavering support, inspiration,
dedication, and love.

and

To my parents,
Julia and Albert,
for everything
I have they made
possible with their
dreams, love, and sacrifice.

ACKNOWLEDGMENTS

• • •

I always dreamed I'd write a book and, even more so, complete one. After practicing women's health for only a short while, I knew I had to put together a simple guide to help women through the menopausal time of life. Now, after nearly twenty years, it's still the case.

As with all challenging and important projects, this one could not have been realized without the help of many people.

First, I would like to thank my great agent Sheree Bykofsky for her diligence, and interest, and Kensington Publishing, for making it possible for all women to access this information.

Thanks also, to:

My collaborator David Green for his unending hard work, encouragement, and enthusiasm for this project.

My very good friend Cheri Whitehead, for her personal insight, editing assistance, and general support.

Eileen Palmer, who helped promote our concepts to the public, and gave me personal strength and loyalty during good times and bad.

The staff of WomanKind Medical Group, past and present, who worked hard to exemplify women's health care at its finest; especially Sylvia Thuet, Anne Isbell, Geri Cunningham, Ana Costa, Heather Steward, and Karen Ripley, who saw me through the last stages of the completion of this book, and all our stressful transitions.

To all my colleagues who inspired me positively and negatively to write this book, and for their guidance in the clinical aspects of it.

I'd like to thank my family for their humor and encouragement.

Most of all, thank you to my loyal patients, who, since 1981, have taught me so much more about menopause, how to adjust therapies, and improve the quality of life than any book that I have ever studied. Their patience, understanding, and keen interest have motivated me to write this book about a poorly understood and very important time of life.

—Joyce A. Kakkis, M.D.

CONTENTS

• • •

INTRODUCTION

● ● ●

Despite its title, this book is not just about estrogen. In a strange way, this book is really about *balance.*

Balance.

It's so hard to achieve in today's society. Even if each of us considers herself to be a balanced individual, there is so much trying to throw us off-balance.

Work. School. Family. The innumerable joys and crises of day-to-day living. Each one pushing, pulling, affecting our balance and our sense of well-being.

Our friends. Our coworkers. The media. Each bringing us pleasure, yet at times, each adding to a daily cacophony of opinions and thoughts.

When it comes to health care, balance is critical. As with the story of Goldilocks, too much and too little are unacceptable. Our goal is to find what's "just right." That's difficult when today's cure is tomorrow's cancer cause, or the old wives' cure of yesteryear turns out to be the wonder drug of the future. Fad diets, fad foods, fad health care, and fad fitness . . . all promising to be "just right," when they so often deliver excess or are sorely lacking.

In the course of writing this book, it was pointed out to me that I might be falling into the same trap. By seeming to promote hormones, and particularly estrogen, I might be contributing to the "one-size-fits-all" mode of thought that pervades our national health debate. It might even seem as though I was promoting estrogen as a cure-all, a one-drug wonder pill that could solve all women's health-care needs.

Nothing could be further from the truth.

Estrogen is not the only answer, but it is, and should be, one of the answers. If we are to achieve a balanced, well-planned, intelligently managed health-care plan for ourselves, it is important for us to understand all the options, and estrogen is one option that must be considered. In fact, it may be said that for many women, estrogen is not optional if good health and peace of mind are to be maintained.

On the other hand, the answer to the true or false statement, "Estrogen is for *everyone*," is a resounding FALSE!

There is no one-way, one-regimen, one-choice approach. You *can* have it your way. In this book, we describe many, many paths you might choose to take, depending on your own individual needs. I am not an estrogen evangelist because I believe estrogen is THE cure-all for anything, but because I feel the need to counter an overwhelming negative portrayal of estrogen in the media and certain parts of the medical community. Left unchecked, this portrayal will deprive women of an option for a balanced and healthy medical regimen through the menopause years and beyond. I'm writing this book because a lot of women avoid estrogen, not because of any perceived risk, but because they are not dealing with a skilled provider who can adjust the dosages and deal with the side effects. Even worse, some women are not making the best choices because they don't have enough information to choose wisely.

The goal of this book is to inform women and guide their decisions, to help take away the guesswork about what's available and what's appropriate. The current media climate seems to be giving a more visible platform to people who are opposed to hormone therapy right now, or we are paying more attention to the negative. Much of the fear and debate over breast implants, the Pill, and other controversial medical topics going back to the 1960s has spilled over into the hormone arena, making people wary of taking anything. Occasional media reports, hints and rumors linking hormones to cancer have instilled in many women a reluctance even to discuss hormone therapy.

This book hopes to fight back, clear the air, and demystify the decision-making process. Whether you choose to take estrogen—natural, synthetic, or herbal—or not, you should make your decision based on sound scientific principles, or know if it's an educated guess. You should know that it's your choice, and in your life, it is okay to change your mind. We're learning more every day, and in the next five to ten years, a tremendous amount of scientific information will help all of us make better-informed decisions, even while it simultaneously confuses us further.

Most women choose not to take estrogen out of fear, poor information, and intolerable side effects. Sometimes, a woman will try estrogen once, have a bad experience, and give up, never to try it again. Health-care providers may have just one chance to treat the patient, and it is critical for us to get the relationship right the first time, so we may endure through the trial period until the dosage is right. Expectations must be set to appropriate levels from the start, and the physician needs to help the patient understand that tuning for the correct dosage may take weeks or even months, and it has to be reevaluated throughout life. I want to help women make the choice based on scientific evidence and personal risk profile. I want to prove to women that dosage adjustment and other "tricks of the trade" can manage side effects, often quite simply.

I want to encourage women to make choices to improve the *quality* of life, as well as the *quantity*. That's an important issue when you look at risk factors. Women who make the hormone decision based purely on fear of cancer may think they are extending the quantity of life, when in fact osteoporosis, memory loss, and heart disease may instead rob their last years of quality, and possibly shorten them as well.

The following statistics on osteoporosis only hint at the effect that estrogen can have on women's life quality:

- Osteoporosis (a progressive loss of bone material that may lead to fractures) affects more than 20 million postmenopausal women in the U.S. alone.[1]
- Bone loss due to osteoporosis results in more than 1.5 million fractures a year in the U.S., including 250,000 hip fractures.[2]
- A 56-year-old white woman has a 15.6 percent lifetime risk

of developing a vertebral fracture, a 16 percent risk of a wrist fracture, and a 17.5 percent risk of hip fracture, and a 40 percent risk that she will experience any of the three during the remainder of her life.[3]
- Hispanic, Asian, and Native American women may be at even greater risk. (African-American women are least at risk for osteoporosis of any group.)[4]
- The direct costs of osteoporosis in the U.S. are estimated at $13.8 billion per year.[5]
- If current trends continue, the prevalence of osteoporosis may double by the year 2020.[6]

Estrogen can slow down the process of bone loss and, alone or in combination with other treatment, may reverse the bone loss that results from osteoporosis. Many of us don't realize that even without fractures, bone loss can be very painful.

Some more statistics:

- Cardiovascular disease is the leading cause of death among women.[7]
- Heart disease kills more women than men and more than all forms of cancer combined. In fact, heart disease kills more women than all cancers, pneumonia, diabetes, and chronic obstructed pulmonary disease (COPD) combined.
- Heart disease kills six to eight times as many women as breast cancer.

Estrogen has been demonstrated to greatly reduce the risk of heart disease in nearly all women, by as much as 50 percent.

Why are there so many books on estrogen out there? Because women are hungry for information. Many of my patients say they have read every hormone-related book available, yet they still ask me for more recommendations. They feel that they still don't have the information they are seeking. Why, then, should you read this book?

Here are a few quick answers:

- It answers the questions the other books don't answer.
- It summarizes, in plain English, information the other books only provide in technical, medical jargon.
- It provides a balanced approach.
- It includes a self-assessment so you can help to determine for yourself if you may be menopausal.
- It clarifies some of the natural versus synthetic options in therapy, and gives dosage options for both.

and, most importantly:

- Many of the other books were not written by professionals who have had nearly twenty years of experience in managing and providing hormone therapy for women of all ages and backgrounds.

I have treated thousands of women with hormones for menopausal, premenopausal, and perimenopausal symptoms. The overwhelming, thunderous appreciation that returns to my office daily lets us know we are doing the *right thing*. We are improving lives, lengthening life spans, and making our patients and their families happier.

A woman today can anticipate living over 80 years—at least 29 years beyond the average menopause and 37 years beyond the average perimenopause. Despite her longer life, she may suffer from a significant number of debilitating illnesses, such as osteoporosis, arthritis, stroke, urinary incontinence, and mental depression, among others. All of these are linked to and influenced by deficiencies of estrogen.

Health is determined by genetics, culture, environmental pollution, exposure to pathogens (illness-causing substances), and lifestyle factors. Many of these influences are beyond our control. Others, we can affect. We cannot afford to be uninformed, when our knowledge can be the only thing that allows us to act, and to manifest some control of our lives, especially our health care.

Women over the age of 60 occupy 40 percent of our hospital

beds and the majority of the nursing home beds. We are living longer but not necessarily better, and we need to make some changes. Our very health and independence is riding on it. The complexity of the aging process in women, particularly the effects of menopause, long and short term, needs to be better understood and better managed; more health-care providers need to receive proper training.

You don't have to believe me. Believe my patients. It is their stories I present in the following pages, their tales of improved health, reduced disease, and more satisfying and productive lives.

WHY THIS BOOK?

●　　●　　●

In my practice as a gynecologist, I see and treat thousands of women a year for a variety of health problems. As the president and medical director of a women's health center, I am also in regular contact with a number of physicians, who, like me, spend their days helping to heal women, to make them healthier, and to enrich our patients' understanding of their own bodies. We have made progress over the years, but we still have a long way to go.

Day after day, there is one thing that bothers me.

Women come to see me, reporting symptoms that include difficulty in concentrating, loss of short-term memory, sleep deprivation, and a number of vaginal and urinary tract complaints—sometimes even abnormal bleeding from the uterus. Many of them also report frequent attacks of intense warmth, which spreads from their faces to their necks and chests, is accompanied by redness and perspiration, and followed by a chill. This disturbing sensation may last up to ten minutes, and happen several times a day.

Often, these women say they are drying up sexually, both literally and figuratively. Their sexual desire has greatly decreased, and no wonder—these patients tell me that their vaginas and vulvas are drying up; the skin is turning pale and thin. When I examine them, I discover that these organs, as well as the urethra, are atrophying, or shrinking, and have become irritated enough to render sexual intercourse painful and even cause bleeding. With some encouragement, a patient may even admit to me that she is having bladder problems—loss of urine with exercise or even ordinary activity—

that cause her to stain her clothing or cause her embarrassment in public places.

As if this frightening set of symptoms were not enough, upon further examination, I might occasionally find that these women also exhibit trouble concentrating, osteoporosis, and cardiovascular disease. With all this, it is no wonder these patients also report being depressed, moody, and irritable.

Yes, seeing these patients is upsetting to me, because frequently, they've already been to several health practitioners and have not been helped—instead, they've been told this is natural and has to be endured. I find that unconscionable, because you see, all of the symptoms I've just described are treatable by a widely known and readily available therapy. In fact, although many of these women have no idea what ails them, my diagnosis is usually very straightforward, easily confirmed, and simply demonstrated to the patient.

Amazingly, some or all of these symptoms I've been describing will strike virtually 100 percent of all women. That's right. If you are a woman (and if you're reading this, that's pretty likely), you will experience some of these health problems, most likely in your early 40s (but possibly as soon as your 30s or even 20s), with the intensity and number of symptoms increasing as you approach your 50s.

That's because the symptoms I've been describing are those of *menopause* and the years surrounding and including menopause, the *perimenopause*.

The really frightening fact?

The treatment I prescribe to my patients is often feared and resisted by them.

The treatment that has so many women worried, although it could literally save their lives? Estrogen.

The hormone estrogen, as part of hormone replacement therapy, or HRT (which may include the addition of the hormones progesterone and/or testosterone), can prevent or even reverse many of the symptoms of menopause and perimenopause. It can extend women's lives and ensure that the quality of the last half of their lives doesn't deteriorate too far. It can reduce pain and disease, increase good health, and enable a longer and more enjoyable sex life. Simply put, hormone replacement therapy can allow a woman to feel good and productive throughout her life and long into the twilight of her life.

Unfortunately, hormone replacement therapy and estrogen have gotten a bad rap. Some doctors and others in the medical community, the media, and other information sources have unfairly pointed to estrogen as being unsafe for all women, when it is not. Estrogen has been named a major cancer risk in some research studies, which again—for *most* women, based on other studies—it is *not.* News stories naming estrogen the culprit in any one of a number of health risk studies often get played up in the news, while those stories touting estrogen's benefits or refuting the studies are sometimes ignored.

Yet day in and day out in my practice, and in the practices of the physicians I work with, we prescribe estrogen. Literally thousands of my patients have been taking it, ever since I first began treating women in the early 1980s. I have prescribed estrogen to young women who could not believe they were perimenopausal at the age of 20, and to retired grandmothers who thought they were too old to be seen buying tampons, and thought taking estrogen meant having periods. I have prescribed it to career women and housewives, married women, single women, and widows. I have prescribed it to women who thought it was "unnatural" to tamper with nature's cycle to prevent menopause, and to those who had seen so many doctors and tried so many other remedies that they were willing to try anything, *anything,* to feel a little better, for a little while.

And the results?

Patient after patient who tells me her life has turned around; who thanks me from the bottom of her heart for returning her health, her lifestyle, and her "sanity." Patients whose family members tell me they can't believe the changes, and most importantly, the improvement. My office receives many letters of praise, not just for our work, but for the therapy itself. Health-center physicians and staff members are frequently stopped in public places to receive heartfelt, unsolicited, and spontaneous testimonials to the efficacy of hormone replacement therapy. The women who stop them often express complete and total amazement that hormone replacement therapy works wonders, and yet they were initially nervous about beginning HRT treatment.

Many of the women who were so concerned, so worried about beginning treatment when they first entered my offices, later call their transformation from sickness to health "miraculous."

Sadly, though, the stigma against estrogen is so strong in some quarters that these same women who are so vocal in my office keep quiet about it with their family and friends for fear of being chastised, lectured, or ridiculed. Instead of spreading the word, they keep it like a secret to themselves, living longer, better, happier lives, while unable to help their own friends, mothers, sisters, and daughters do the same. I notice a remarkable similarity to the old fears of the birth-control pill shortly after it was introduced. Now, of course, we know the Pill provides many health benefits, but at the time, widespread and often erroneous reports of side effects kept many women from even considering it.

Simply put, *all* women benefit from estrogen, but not all women can or will take it, because it must be balanced against risk. The questions we need to ask are how much to give, in what form to give it, when, and for how long. It may be all-natural or synthetic. It may be combined with other hormones in a multifaceted regimen. The risk-to-benefit ratio is the critical point of decision. In most cases, the benefit far outweighs the risk, but as with all prevention, it takes imagination to see future problems before they become reality.

Unfortunately, the ability of women to make a decision on whether or not to take estrogen is often deterred by an overload of biased, inaccurate, and incomplete information. There are many books—written by doctors who do not practice hormone therapy, non-doctors who do not have medical knowledge, and others who just have no place commenting on the subject—books that mislead and frighten women. Some of these books become popular enough that their misinformation becomes "common knowledge," sometimes even accepted by doctors who should know better but do not have access to more rigorously presented medical information. Other books have been very helpful and started the trend of quality information for women. Reading a variety of opinions is better than trusting one source.

Several years ago, I finally reached the point where I realized that merely treating my patients was not enough. I needed to do some preaching. I needed to stand on a mountaintop and shout to the world. Testify. Create a new Estrogen Gospel to replace the old one, and lead women to a postmenopausal Promised Land.

So I've become an Estrogen Evangelist.

Like all evangelism, it is hard work. Slow and steady work. One person at a time work. It is work that at some times requires urgency, and at others requires extreme caution. It is work that can be both brain numbingly tedious and frighteningly fast-paced. It is also work that can be gratifying and rewarding in a nearly spiritual manner. The methodology by which I acquire converts is simple: Take women who are menopausal and let them judge for themselves as the hormone replacement therapy improves their moods, heals their bodies, increases well-being, sharpens their minds, and heightens their sexuality. Take women who are perimenopausal, and let them "feel the power" as estrogen strips away the symptoms one at a time, letting them feel almost as though they have stopped some of the negative aspects of aging, as the effects of advancing menopause are stopped in their tracks.

This is not a book about general physiology or anatomy. This book is about the specifics of the menopause, the specifics of hormone replacement therapy, and the specifics of properly educating women dealing with these issues so they can make informed choices. It is a book women can use to identify their own symptoms and challenges with menopause and hormone replacement therapy.

I am an Estrogen Evangelist. These are my confessions. This book is my gospel.

Read on.

The Gospel Truth

• • •

As you read this book, there may be times when you just don't want to read the entire chapter. Maybe you don't think it applies to you. Maybe you just don't have the time. So, at the end of each chapter, I've summarized the key points in a section called "The Gospel Truth." If you just want to breeze through this book and get a quick overall understanding of the issues involving estrogen, or if you've read the book and want to refresh your memory about the key facts, you may do so by reading "The Gospel Truth" for each section.

2

MENOPAUSE
Natural—Or Is It?

● ● ●

Given the symptoms discussed in the previous chapter, you can see why the menopause can be a very confusing and upsetting time of life for many women. Although some women are fortunate enough to pass through it with seemingly few signs, symptoms, or disruption, many women suffer serious physical, emotional, and mental disturbances.

The median age of menopause is 51, but the actual age at which a woman may reach the "change of life" varies greatly. Typically, it begins between ages 40 and 45 and virtually all women have experienced symptoms by age 52. Some unfortunate women suffer hormonal dysfunction and loss of estrogen as early as their teens. Others are lucky enough to make it into their 90s with few significant symptoms. However, not having symptoms does not mean changes are not occurring. Over the years, women's menstrual periods have started at a younger and younger age, while the average age of menopause has not changed much.

The causes of menopause or other estrogen deficiencies are usually "natural" or genetically determined, but can also be from disruptions such as injury, surgery, chemotherapy, radiation, and other toxic agents. Even stress, if severe enough, can halt ovarian function and estrogen production. All the causes may be assisted by environmental and lifestyle factors. For example, it appears that thinner women and smokers enter the change a little sooner. In fact, smoking seems to lower the body's estrogen in general.

The popular perception is that menopause begins when the

menstrual periods stop. Technically, this is true: Menopause is defined as "the permanent cessation of menses that occurs after the end of ovarian function." In actuality, though, the years before and decades after the cessation of bleeding are of greater clinical significance than menopause itself. The period before menopause, also called the perimenopause, can begin seven to eight years before menopause. It is often signaled with signs and symptoms—a common one being variations in the menstrual cycle, which can become more frequent or less frequent, too heavy or too light or just different. Remember: Periods cannot be distinguished from other bleeding. Some women experience periods that are brown, black, sticky, or bright red with heavy clots, all of which can be a normal variation. Depression, moodiness, and hot flashes can also happen during this time, even though the actual menopause has not occurred yet. These changes can be like "circling the drain" for those who have serious symptoms, or merely a confusing time for others.

There are actually several definitions of perimenopause, depending upon whom you speak to. Many people believe menopause is only one day in a woman's life, confirmed when she has not had a period for 12 consecutive months, or when menopause is induced via surgery, illness, or other artificial means. Perimenopause is sometimes defined as 6 years or more prior, and 1 year after the period stops.[8] The entire experience may last as long as 10 years. The distinction between perimenopause, postmenopause, and menopause is somewhat arbitrary—most women consider the entire experience "menopause," whether many years or few.

Menopause before 40 is usually considered premature menopause, and if natural, may be genetic and indicate a potential problem with the immune system. Women who experience premature menopause are at increased risk for osteoporosis and heart disease,[9] because they lack estrogen for a longer period of time, if untreated. Sometimes, even adolescents can experience a type of menopause due to an excessive exercise program, low body weight, eating disorders, and other related circumstances. This type of menopause is usually temporary, and responds to lifestyle change, but deficiencies still must be treated, because these girls are at the same risk from the low-estrogen state and its related problems and symptoms as older women. The reality is, menopause is premature anytime it happens before you expect it or want it, and it's late anytime it happens later than you had in mind. (Believe it or not, some women positively anticipate the onset of menopause. For example, a woman may have fibroids, and may hope the menopause will help shrink them. Or they may simply prefer to be part of the crowd—just as when your periods first started, you felt left out if some of you started sooner than the majority.)

It is estimated that 75 percent of perimenopausal women in the U.S. have hot flashes. As many at 85 percent experience varying degrees of trouble during menopause for at least one year. And 25 percent of women have problems for more than five years. More than 30 percent of the female population in the United States is postmenopausal, and this percentage is increasing as the Baby Boom generation enters its 50s and beyond.

We are fortunate to live in a time when medical technology and pharmaceuticals have extended our life spans far beyond that of our ancestors. Unfortunately, though, our longer lives exceed the design of our bodies, which were created initially to last about 45 years. Statistics from the U.S. Department of Health and Human Services show that women are living far longer than in the past— American women's life spans increased from 58.7 years in 1929 to 78.9 years in 1995. That's a 20-year increase in just 70 years! And as life spans lengthen and Baby Boomers age, the number of women between the ages of 45 and 64 increases commensurately. The U.S. population of 45-to-64-year-olds is expected to rise from 52 million in 1995 to 71 million in 2005 to over 85 million in 2050! With these record numbers of women experiencing menopause, we could encounter a different type of "global warming" not predicted by the environmentalists!

In the past, death soon followed the birth of a woman's last child, while today's woman can expect to live well into her 80s. To put it in perspective, on the average today, a woman lives about a third of her life after menopause, and in some cases, it's nearer to half her life; indeed, the number of years a woman lives after menopause may exceed the number of years she lived before it!

Postmenopausal life has become a significant portion of a woman's life span, and it is incumbent upon both physicians and patients to improve the quality of these years, not just the number. Women's bodies were never intended to last 30 to 40 years in an estrogen-deficient state. The concept that it is "natural" and therefore good to avoid hormonal intervention is somewhat of a misnomer, and we must make adjustments in our perceptions to accommodate a more realistic view.

Each woman's response to the medical and psychological manifestations of menopause may be different. Proper therapy requires consideration not only for a woman's hormonal status and the possibility of replacement, but also an overall "whole-woman" evaluation, including her cardiovascular, bone, mental, and spiritual health. Since many other changes are occurring for women at this time of life—such as increased frequency of major diseases, separation from or difficulties with children, loss of or illness of parents, loss or illness of spouse, relationship changes, and often divorce—it is important to take these issues into account when deciding how best to manage the patient's symptoms, many of which may be aggravated by stress. Hormone replacement therapy (HRT) is designed to replace these hormones that are no longer produced by a woman's body, in a gentle and gradual fashion, diminishing or even eliminating the effects of perimenopause and menopause.

Some of the changes resulting from estrogen loss occur slowly. It has taken medical science many years to demonstrate both the risks of deficiency and the problems of excess in hormonal levels. The convoluted interweaving of the hormones estrogen, progesterone, and testosterone with the multiple organs of the body, including the uterus and breasts, makes it a complex and difficult area of study, requiring more diligent research and carefully gathered information. Even if we do not know all, we do know a great deal more at this point than we did in the past. Individualization of the therapy has emerged as critical to success, in determining when and how to intervene, as well as monitoring patients once intervention has begun. Regardless of the information both pro and con, each woman has to make her own choice and once that choice is made, she should be flexible in changing that choice if the circumstances in her life change such as to warrant it. Most importantly, no woman should be made to feel guilty about her choice, whether for or against. The availability of full, accurate information is the key to a woman's being able to make an intelligent choice for herself.

The importance of this need for full, accurate information becomes even more obvious when one considers: Since the estrogen-related cancer scares of the late 1970s, much research has been done, the doses have been modified and reduced drastically, and many of the risks have been reduced via such techniques as cycling estrogen with progesterone or progestin, and using non-oral doses to localize the effects of the hormone. Estrogen is much safer now than it was when it burst into widespread use in the 1960s, but the spread of information has not kept up with the improvements.

Unfortunately, studies reveal that many menopausal women are still afraid to take hormones. Less than 7 percent of menopausal patients under the care of an internist take hormone replacement therapy; for those being treated for menopause by an obstetrician/gynecologist, the figure is about 23 percent. Despite all the reasons I've detailed for trying hormone replacement therapy in general, and estrogen specifically, it is estimated that over 50 percent of all menopausal women are not using it at all. The reasons most often cited, are fear, lack of symptoms, or that it was never offered to them.

The fear is typically fear of cancer, particularly uterine and breast cancer. Slightly lower on the list is fear of side effects. Even for women who eventually try estrogen, this fear makes compliance with the therapy difficult. After starting therapy, a woman may encounter strong negative reaction from friends and family who may discourage her from continuing. Combined with the occasional side effect that does happen, this negative influence may persuade her to give up. What makes it worse is that some doctors may not make a woman aware of all the possible treatment options, so she may give up on treatment entirely instead of trying another form of treatment with less risk or fewer side effects. Both the cancer risk and risk of side effects can be greatly reduced and managed through proper therapy.

When we balance the choices, estrogen may be beneficial for most but *not all* women. I respect the decision to take or not to take hormones equally, as long as the facts were presented and understood when the decision was made. Surprised?

The Gospel Truth—MENOPAUSE: Natural—Or Is It?

• • •

1. The median age of menopause is 51, but may vary from the teen years to the late 50s in extreme cases.
2. Menopause can be defined as the "the end of periods," but the onset of the perimenopause may begin seven to eight years prior.
3. Perimenopause is defined as the transitional years prior to menopause and one year after. It may last as long as 10 years.
4. More than 30 percent of the female population of the United States is postmenopausal.
5. Menopause before 40 is considered premature menopause.
6. During menopause and perimenopause the production of the hormones estrogen, progesterone and testosterone tapers off.
7. Hormone replacement therapy (HRT) is designed to replace the hormones that are no longer produced by a woman's body.
8. Menopause often occurs during a time of other great changes in a woman's life. These issues may both mask and exacerbate symptoms of menopause, confusing self-awareness of the condition.

9. Today's woman can expect to live 80 or more years, meaning she may spend at least a third of her life after menopause. Women's bodies may not have been designed to function 30 to 40 years without estrogen and other related hormones.

10. Individualization of estrogen replacement therapy is critical to its successful use.

3

TOOLS FOR EVALUATION
Obtaining a Meaningful Confession

● ● ●

I may be an evangelist, but I'm not a psychic. Like any physician, I depend upon my patients to describe their symptoms to me before I can begin treatment. With menopause, however, the symptoms can be a little ambiguous . . . fuzzy . . . so rather than a list of symptoms, many times, my patients will tell me stories—their stories. Sometimes, all it takes is a simple little story of a symptom here, a symptom there, and I can begin putting together the puzzle, and attempt to develop a plan of treatment. Other times, it's a bit harder. I need to delve deeply. This process takes somewhat longer, but I've come up with a system that makes it more successful and easier for both of us. I don't want patients to feel like they're confessing to a crime when they've come in for a simple visit to the doctor!

How do I know if a patient's "time of change" has begun? My method of evaluation makes the best of the physician-patient interaction. It begins with a very important component: listening. Physicians cannot help their patients by doing all the talking. Listening and responding in an open-minded, logical, and nonjudgmental manner is very important. Easy to say, but harder to accomplish than you might imagine. We, as women's health practitioners, want to protect our patients from harm and implement therapy to prevent bone loss and accelerated heart disease, while delivering many other health benefits. In our rush to protect, we have to listen to what the patient's immediate needs are and build these into the start of our solution. The patient's priority must be addressed while we paint the whole picture.

As a woman coming to a professional for help, you must become a willing partner in providing information in a straightforward, honest fashion. For this purpose, my practice uses a hormonal journal that is very useful for the patient, the physician, and other health-care providers. *(See Appendix C.)*

All of the symptoms listed in the journal are clues. Everyone knows about hot flashes, but the patient may not realize the correlation between menopause and symptoms such as memory loss, bone and joint pain, irritability, and sleep disturbances. Putting together her medical history, the interview, and the journal creates a picture of where she is.

After a thorough interview, a physical examination will be done, sometimes in the same sitting, sometimes at a later appointment. The symptoms of menopause could also exist for other reasons, which must be identified or eliminated as well. But there are many physical hints of hormone insufficiency—dry skin, vaginal dryness, pale genital tissues, and breast tenderness, among others—that help substantiate the condition. Pap smears are taken as well, and can be analyzed for estrogen effect in the body.

Blood may also be drawn, since blood levels of follicle stimulating hormone or FSH (which increases when estrogen is low), estrogen itself, and support hormones such as testosterone, thyroid, and progesterone can all be helpful in determining a hormonal baseline. Lab tests may be done to establish a level of confidence that estrogen deficiency exists, even if the clinical signs are clear. The drawback, however, is that lab tests are not always an accurate depiction of hormone deficiency; levels may vary depending on when blood was drawn, sensitivity differences, and any medication taken. If tests are positive, they are generally reliable, but when negative, they do not necessarily eliminate the possibility of the condition. The day of the menstrual cycle on which the sample is drawn may affect the test results and is a very important factor to consider. The symptoms a woman expresses and the progression of them are far more important than any of the objective scientific measures. Women know their own bodies: If we listen, they will help diagnose themselves.

Another important tool for evaluation is pelvic ultrasound, which can help determine the cause of bleeding irregularities. (This test bounces sound waves off the internal organs and creates a picture.) These irregularities are very common, and we have to separate normal menopausal bleeding (or lack thereof) from other potential problems or conditions, such as fibroids, polyps, and precancerous uterine problems.

Once we have the history, physical exam, desired lab results, and other related tests, we can custom-design the hormone replacement. "Regimen base"—the appropriate dosages that work best for you—will be subject to change and monitoring in the first year, until we achieve a close-to-perfect balance of symptom control, health protection, and side-effect elimination. It will then need periodic reevaluation throughout your life to recognize benefits and limit risks.

Salivary hormone tests use fluid collected from your mouth to evaluate hormone levels. The results may be correlated with blood serum levels, but an understanding as to what level creates the physiologically desired effect is still not clear. It is yet to be determined, for example, what salivary progesterone level clearly protects the lining of the uterus from cancerous change.

Salivary analysis can be done of estrogen, progesterone, testosterone, and other hormone levels, and can be a useful adjunct to hormone supervision. It has the advantage of avoiding a blood test. The most important thing, however, is to stick to one type of measurement. Just as when comparing your weight, it helps to use the same scale and weigh at the same time of day, you should monitor your hormone levels by one consistent method. Hopping from one type of analysis to another is not useful.

Who Are the Hormone Players?

There are four main hormones that are of primary interest in a woman's midlife analysis: Estrogen, progesterone, testosterone, and thyroid hormone.

Estrogen is a "female" hormone that is produced by multiple organs in a woman's body, but primarily by the ovaries. Age, as well as different environmental or physical stresses, may cause estrogen production to decrease, increase, or cease altogether. During pregnancy, for example, estrogen levels are actually boosted and have a relative fall in the postpartum period. This hormone is the one primarily responsible for the buildup of the lining of the uterus that ultimately sheds with our period and that maintains the moisture in our mucous membranes and skin, the quality of our hair and nails, and multiple other important functions, including mental function.

There are several types of estrogen: estrone (E1), estradiol (E2), and estriol (E3). Of the three, estriol is the weakest. Estrone is the estrogen most thought to be linked to greater risk of breast cancer. Estrogen therapies may contain one, two, or all three estrogens. The safety and effectiveness of all three types is not clearly understood.

Progesterone, which is also primarily female, is the hormone responsible for the shedding of the lining of the uterus after estrogen has built it up, creating our period. Progestin and progestogen are compounds that act like progesterone in the body; all three terms are often used interchangeably. (There are scientific differences that won't concern us for the purposes of this book.) Too much or too little progesterone can contribute to premenstrual syndrome (PMS). Inappropriate progesterone levels can have other side effects and symptoms, including depression and sluggishness. By "inappropriate," I do not necessarily mean "low": The effect of hormones is more dependent on their delicate balance in the body than the simple fact of having them or not having them.

The combination of estrogen and progesterone in balance in the body maintains the integrity and health of the uterus and other organs.

Testosterone plays a role in the resilience of vaginal and vulvar tissues and in feelings of well-being. This primarily "male" hormone or *androgen* is produced in small amounts by a woman's ovaries, adrenal glands, liver, fat cells, and skin. When an ovary is removed or goes through menopausal change, the relative balance of testosterone is changed. Testosterone is replaced primarily in order to restore lost *libido,* or sexual desire, in women. Overreplacement causes male effects such as hair growth, voice changes, acne, irritability, or hostile behavior.

Lastly, *thyroid* hormone should be evaluated and checked periodically throughout a woman's life. Both deficiency and extra production of this hormone occur frequently and can cause significant trouble. Low thyroid is associated with fatigue, slow reflexes, dry skin and hair, difficulty with concentration, cold intolerance, and other irregularities. It can also make it appear as if your cholesterol is high. Excess thyroid is associated with nervousness, irritability, rapid heartbeat, difficulty concentrating, and sleep disturbances. It is a relatively easy hormone to assess and replace, and should be part of a woman's initial screening for problems in midlife. Since thyroid hormone can "confuse" the symptoms of menopause, it should certainly be a part of a woman's hormonal evaluation and general wellness check. (Many of us "hope" for thyroid problems, to explain weight gain and provide a simple treatment for weight loss, but the answer is not always so easy. Thyroid problems carry their own set of complications, and are not something to be wished for!)

Although these four hormones have significant impact on our proper functioning, the general backdrop of the body's overall physiology is still very important. Other factors that need to be considered when the change of life is being evaluated include triglycerides and lipid balance in the blood, anemia, urinary tract infection, cholesterol, sugar balance, and calcium, magnesium, and other minerals. Heart disease and osteoporosis must also be aggressively monitored and treated, because the consequences of ignoring these conditions are dire.

The following chapters tell the stories of some of the many women whom I've treated. These are women who came to me when they needed help . . . and they expected it from me. I listened to their stories; I read their journals; and I did what I could, often with tremendous results. I did not always succeed. Sometimes I had to try again and again—but I don't give up easily. Keep the processes I've described in mind as you read on and explore these women's experiences, which may be like your own, or those of someone you know.

The Gospel Truth—TOOLS FOR EVALUATION: Obtaining a Meaningful Confession

• • •

1. Truly listening and responding to patients in an open-minded, logical, and nonjudgmental manner is an important part of a doctor's medical evaluation.

2. A hormonal journal may help patients, doctors, and other health-care providers come to a greater awareness of the symptoms the patient is experiencing and the interrelationship of the symptoms.

3. Lab tests, while not definitive, may help corroborate and explain the symptoms a woman reports.

4. Helpful tests for hormone evaluation include blood and salivary tests. It is important to stick with one type of test and to test at the same time in the menstrual cycle, to get meaningful results.

5. Estrogen is the primary female hormone responsible for changes in a woman's midlife.

6. The three types of estrogen are: estrone (E1), estradiol (E2), and estriol (E3). Estrogen therapy may contain one, two, or all three types.

7. Progesterone plays a large role in reducing the risk of uterine cancer for women who are taking estrogen therapy.

8. Testosterone is a "male" hormone that is also needed by some women. It influences sex drive and is normally produced by the ovary.

9. Thyroid hormone is responsible for preventing fatigue, maintaining reflexes, and preventing dry skin and hair. Lack of hormone may cause difficulty concentrating, cold intolerance, weight gain, and other irregularities.

10. These hormones are important, but must be considered along with evaluations for cholesterol, triglycerides, anemia, urinary tract infection, sugar balance, and calcium, magnesium, and other minerals, as well as heart and bone health.

HOT FLASHES
"I Have Hot Flashes, But I Still Have My Period, So I Can't Be Menopausal."

• • •

Kate, a 48-year-old executive of a local company, told me:

"You're the fifth doctor I've been to this year, and I'm having a problem with what I think are hot flashes. They happen mostly at night, but they happen sometimes in the day as well. I'll find myself tossing the covers off at night, and my partner will be freezing. In the office where I work, I keep turning the thermostat down, and everyone complains that they're too cold. Sometimes I wake up with a sweat that soaks my hair, pillow, and nightclothes. I'm not imagining these soaking episodes, and they're ruining my sleep. The most annoying thing is that I'm an executive of a large company, and it appears that I can trigger these flashes by stress, such as when I get up in front of a big group to give a presentation. It's very embarrassing for me, and I need help. The last doctors I saw told me that because my periods have not gone away, I can't be menopausal, and they refuse to consider a hormone evaluation or treat me."

Both lay people and professionals have a black-and-white understanding of menopause. For many people, the attitude toward menopause seems to be "either you are or you're not menopausal."

Simply put, this is wrong.

Menopause is a continuum. Starting with the menopausal

transition, which begins 7 to 8 years before the actual cessation of menstruation, and continuing with the perimenopausal years following that, the entire menopause "envelope" is something that transcends and belies such a black-and-white approach.

The "hot flash," also called "hot flush" (or, more recently, a "power surge"), is just one sign of encroaching or full-fledged menopause. Technically called vasomotor symptoms, hot flashes usually begin as a warm feeling in a localized area of the upper body (such as the neck, chest, or face), and spread out, sometimes over the entire body. The skin may turn red, and you may break into a sweat.

But if, as it's been said, there are 50 ways to leave your lover, there are at least a hundred ways to have a hot flash. Here are a few:

- Sweating on the chest
- Sweating on top of the head
- Heat or sweating behind the knees
- Sweating of the feet
- Hot sensation followed by a cold chill
- Profuse sweating just from the temples
- Heat starting at the chest and moving up to the forehead
- Hot hands
- Sweating in the middle of the low back
- Heat in any part of the body without any sweat at all

Many people assume that hot flashes are just a sensation, but the body's temperature is actually rising—skin temperature may rise as much as 7 degrees! If you can imagine being outside on a 105-degree day, wearing all your clothes, you can imagine what it's like to have a hot flash.

In some cases, women perspire so profusely they waken to soaked bedclothes and bedsheets. Hot flashes may be so intense or so frequent that a woman becomes hesitant to leave her home. Hot flashes may occur rarely—indeed, some women never experience them—or they may occur as much as every few minutes for some women, especially on bad days.

Many women may not realize at first that external influences can and do trigger hot flashes. Hot-flash activators include:

- hot days or warm environments
- hot or spicy food
- stress
- hot beverages
- alcohol
- caffeine

In other words, if you like to start each day in your hectic job at the steel smelter by washing down a breakfast burrito with a big, hot cup of coffee, you may be in serious trouble! On the other hand, women who avoid all the activators on the list may *still* get hot flashes. Women who live in very cold climates are as susceptible as those living in the Sun Belt.

While many women find it possible to cope with daytime hot flashes if not too frequent, those that occur at night can have far-reaching effects. By disturbing sleep—often chronically—night flashes can lower mental sharpness, depress mood, negatively affect job performance, and disrupt relationships. Over the long term, the lack of sleep may cause memory lapses and decreased motor skills, leading to a higher risk of auto accidents, household accidents such as falls and burns, and other seemingly unrelated consequences. (Curiously, even without hot flashes or sweats at night, menopausal women frequently experience severe sleep disturbances, with frequent awakenings through the night.)

Despite the prevalence of the hot-flash and related symptoms, there is no one set of symptoms that makes the diagnosis of menopause. Because it is a continuum, a woman could be having some symptoms but not others. While some women cease menstruating but otherwise exhibit few menopausal symptoms, others continue menstruating—perhaps erratically—while their bodies become textbook cases of the worst effects of menopause. There is little rhyme or reason to it; it's merely a demonstration of the ways that different bodies, different genes, and different environments react to the gradual reduction and eventual loss of estrogen production in the body.

Just as many people erroneously think, "If I'm having hot flashes I'm definitely in menopause," others will aver, "I'm 38 (or 43 or 47) so I'm definitely too young to be in menopause." It's true:

Those *are* relatively young years for a woman to begin feeling the symptoms. In our society, a hot flash is often the laugh-getting symptom of sitcom grandmothers, or—closer to home—the worrisome agent of nighttime discomfort and sleep deprivation experienced by our own mothers. As we've noted, the average age for menopause in the U.S. is 51. But as with all averages, that single number reveals only a small fraction of the story. On either side of that "typical" peak in the statistical curve is a much more relevant story: the great number of women who begin menopause much earlier or later. Just as there are women who do not experience symptoms of the menopause until their 70s, there are those who may experience symptoms in their 20s.

When I encounter an uncommonly young woman who seems to be showing signs of menopause, I test for hormone levels. More often than not, the results do indicate a deficiency, which is confirmed by the treatment: a brief "trial run" using appropriate doses of hormones, which eliminates many or all of the symptoms. The wisdom of the trial run is that the tests, of course, may not tell the whole story, and the trial gives direct feedback, if carefully done.

Now, why do we say that a woman who is still menstruating may be menopausal? A period by any other name may not be a period.

There is no doubt that it is confusing to a woman to be told that she is menopausal when she is still having her period. However, menstruation does not necessarily contraindicate menopausal symptoms, nor does other uterine bleeding distinguish itself from a real period.

Many women lose their periods as the very last thing to happen in their menopausal transition. It is as if the body is a factory being shut down in a very orderly fashion. The hormonal conveyor belts are gradually shut down, the ovarian workers check out for the day, and the last egg out of the office turns off the lights and locks the ovarian door.

Sometimes, though, the last few workers linger, and the nearly closed factory turns out a few last periods, and puts out a random egg or two. (Thus the "surprise" late-life babies.) Hormone-level testing confirms that the factory is obviously not operating at full productivity, but still, those last few periods are a source of doubt and confusion. What exactly is going on?

There are several factors that may be at work when a woman's period seems to be continuing despite other menopausal symptoms. For example, a true period cannot be distinguished from abnormal bleeding. The perimenopausal years are prone to any number of stimuli for abnormal bleeding, such as side effects from polyps, fibroids, stress, and precancerous or cancerous changes.

Or there may simply be enough hormones to trigger a period, but not enough to keep all the body's systems in balance. Remember, many organs contribute to background hormone activity in the body, even though the ovaries are not functioning well. Most women will see changes of some sort in their periods. They will become noticeably further apart or closer. Their ovarian reserve is falling, but has not reached zero.

Women should not take the existence of a period in light of other symptoms of menopause to mean that the menopause is not really happening. It well could be. There is no reason to continue suffering while we wait for an arbitrary event to occur.

Hormone therapy can be just as helpful at this stage as it is afterward in reducing the effect of hot flashes and the other symptoms. It is important to adjust (titrate) carefully the dosage slowly from a very low starting point in order to identify the minimum dosage required for symptom control. Also, it is easier to go up in dosage than get side effects and have to go down. This approach is more comfortable for most women.

Remember our patient Kate, the executive with hot flashes? She just started on low-dose, cyclic replacement therapy. Premarin®, 0.3mg daily was chosen, which represents about 50 percent of the average dose used. Progesterone (Provera®), in 2.5mg doses, was added for 10 days a month. (The progesterone was given on a schedule that imitates the body's normal cycle calendar.) Both of these were advised in the evening, since her symptoms were primarily at night. She experienced complete remission from temperature disturbances and no longer dissolves into a puddle during public presentations. It is likely that she'll require increased doses as the natural background hormone activity continues to wane in her body. Kate was originally concerned that Premarin is derived from pregnant mare's urine, as she had heard that the horses were mistreated. Our investigation did not substantiate these claims, but I feel this decision should be made on an individual basis, and I respect any woman who chooses not to take it.

The Gospel Truth—HOT FLASHES: "I Have Hot Flashes, But I Still Have My Period, So I Can't Be Menopausal."

• • •

1. Hot flashes (also called hot flushes or power surges) are a common and most recognized symptom of menopause.
2. A hot flash usually begins as a warm feeling in the upper body, then spreads out; it can appear in many other variations as well. The body's surface temperature may actually rise several degrees.
3. Hot flashes may or may not be accompanied by sweating. Those that occur at night often disturb sleep.
4. Because menopause is a continuum and varies from individual to individual, a woman may have some symptoms and not others.
5. Menopause can happen prematurely. Though uncommon, it is possible to start having symptoms as early as 20.
6. A woman may be perimenopausal even if she is still having menstrual bleeding.
7. Abnormal bleeding cannot be easily distinguished from a normal period, especially if it occurs at regular intervals.
8. Low-dose hormone therapy is sometimes all that is needed to rebalance a younger woman in the early perimenopause.

5

HEREDITY
"My Mother Sailed Through It."

● ● ●

Linda, a housewife with two children and just recently married for the second time, told me:

"I came to your office today because I'm having a very hard time with my 'change of life.' I've been talking to my mom about it, and she doesn't know why I'm having such a problem. As she remembers it, she and my grandma went through it naturally, with no problem whatsoever. I feel silly and somewhat incompetent because I am having a hard time. Is this psychological on my part? Or am I just oversensitive to the symptoms that I'm experiencing? I tried to talk to my grandmother about it, but she really doesn't remember any detail. Everyone seems to think all I need to do is relax or see a shrink. I thought that was the advice for when you couldn't get pregnant! I drink green tea, eat tofu, exercise, do yoga, take vitamins, yadda yadda yadda, and there's no relief in sight."

Often, a woman's impression that her mother "sailed through" menopause is based on her mother's faulty memory, as well as what her mother may or may not be willing to share with her. How likely is it that mothers who went through the menopause 20 to 30 years ago, have an accurate memory of what it was like? In addition, depending on the era, or community attitude, it may not have been socially acceptable to discuss it, or to admit to suffering from it.

Another factor to consider is that the mother is likely to have gone through menopause when the daughter was in her teens, a time when the daughter is unlikely to have been aware of what was happening, or to understand it even if she was. Furthermore, that is precisely the time when conflicts between daughters and mothers tend to be most acute. Tension from that time may be remembered as stemming from one party's adolescence rather than the other's menopause. Other stresses common to midlife, such as divorce, career change, or depression, may also contribute to a mother's minimizing of menopausal difficulties.

The effects of menopause are easy to sweep under the carpet, and even easier to forget about years later, just as the trauma and "horror stories" of difficult childbirth tend to soften over time.

Other factors make it difficult to link mothers' and daughters' menopausal histories. Genetically speaking, there is a correlation between the age the mother has menopause and the age the daughter does. In today's medical environment, hysterectomies and other non-natural causes of the menopause, such as surgery, make it difficult to have a history that can be traced. A woman may discover she doesn't have any family history to refer to because no one in her family has experienced a natural menopause.

Even when a woman is fortunate enough to have ready access to her family's menopausal history, it may not tell her what to expect. There may be areas of similarity between the mothers' and daughters' experience, and areas of difference. For example, a daughter may begin menopause at the same age as her mother, but she may have night sweats and hot flashes, where her mother didn't.

There are multiple complicating environmental factors as well. General health, exercise, diet, alcohol use, smoking, climate, and stress all affect the onset and intensity of menopausal symptoms. For a number of reasons, a woman today can expect to begin menopause somewhat later than her grandmother did, but then it depends on your definition of "start." Strangely, there seems to be no reproducible correlation between menstruation itself and menopause: Neither the age of menarche (first period), the age at which you become sexually active, nor the number of children you have has a perfectly predictable effect on menopause. Some trends exist; for example, early starters (who have a first period before age 10) are late quitters and late starters are early quitters. . . . Go figure.

Also, while the immediate ancestors in your family tree are important, so are other female relatives. We don't know all the linkages that may contribute to a woman's menopausal tendencies and makeup. Your father's mother, grandmothers, sisters, and other female members of his family, if any, may provide some useful clues as to your menopausal experience and expectations. There have not been enough extensive studies to provide any useful conclusions to date.

Of course, rare and exceptional as they may be, there *are* some women who do, or did, just sail through menopause. This is not to say that the silent, potentially damaging physiological changes did not occur. It is up to the daughters of these fortunate women to acknowledge their mothers' good luck, without taking any mantle or burden of behaving a certain way upon themselves. Regardless of her mother's experience, each woman must make the decision of how to handle her menopause for herself, based on her body, her medical needs, and her personal choices.

Remember Linda, the woman whose mother claimed to just sail through menopause? She just completed 12 months of low-dose treatment with Estrace (a plant-based natural estrogen) and no progesterone because of her history of a prior hysterectomy. Her symptoms are 90 percent improved—her journal continues to show steady progress. She is doing so well she makes entries in her journal very infrequently now, which generally in my experience means the woman is feeling better. She also adopted a walking program and takes vitamins and minerals on a regular schedule. The ongoing support of positive health habits and reevaluation of her hormone needs is the key to estrogen success.

The Gospel Truth—HEREDITY: "My Mother Sailed Through It"

• • •

1. Your mother probably did not sail through it! It's most likely a mistaken impression based upon faulty memory, a misinterpretation of events at the time, and/or historical, social, and cultural biases.
2. If a mother is going through menopause when a daughter is in her teens, tension in the household may more likely be blamed on the teen's "raging" hormones than the mother's diminishing ones.
3. Midlife events, such as divorces, career changes, and children leaving home or going through adolescence may distract women from acknowledging their menopausal symptoms.
4. Mothers and daughters may experience menopause differently, even if they begin it at relatively the same age. If the mother had a hysterectomy, her "unnatural" menopause may have been so different from her daughter's they may be virtually unable to compare the two.
5. Environmental factors such as general health, exercise, diet, smoking, alcohol use, climate, and stress may all affect the onset and intensity of menopausal symptoms.
6. Sometimes, on occasion, a woman does "just sail" through menopause. It does not mean her daughter will—or vice versa. It does not mean the silent damage of osteoporosis and heart disease do not exist.

6

LIFE WITHOUT ESTROGEN
"I Prefer Aging the 'Natural' Way."

● ● ●

Janice, a 44-year-old aerobics instructor and data entry operator at a small graphic design firm, told me:

"It's very important to me that you understand I am very health-oriented. The more natural, the better, as far as I'm concerned. I barely take even an aspirin, and if I can avoid it, I don't take even that. I don't eat red meat; I've exercised regularly since I was a teenager. I had natural childbirth with my two children, and as I face the menopause, I absolutely 100 percent want to do only what's natural. In my heart, I would prefer to treat it with nutrition, exercise intervention, and spiritual and psychological support. The problem is, I'm just not doing well, despite a great deal of effort on my part. I'm having trouble sleeping, my energy level is poor, and my sex drive is zip. I'm here to see if there's some natural therapy with hormones that I can be comfortable about taking. It goes without saying that the lowest dose possible is what I want."

What is natural?

If you were a diabetic, you would seek treatment. It is probable your doctor would prescribe insulin, which is a hormone, and you would take it, because not doing so would endanger your life. Your body, which should normally produce insulin, and had stopped for "natural" reasons, would go into diabetic shock without the vital hormone. It is very likely you would die without it.

You wouldn't *not* take insulin.

So why is it that because estrogen is a female hormone, it is considered elective? Some form of gender bias is at work.

A woman whose body does not produce estrogen is subject to all of the side effects and complications we've been discussing. Some of these conditions, notably heart disease and osteoporosis, are life-threatening, yet often initially silent. Still, some people believe that a woman whose body has stopped producing estrogen should not consider hormone therapy merely because it is not "natural."

As a society, we are liable to fall prey to a preconceived notion that not intervening in physiological changes is natural. Perhaps it is a reaction to spectacular news stories: revelations of unnecessary medical treatment, drugs and other therapies that do more harm than good, invasive and unnecessary surgery, class action suits against pharmaceutical and other medical companies. This reaction against unregulated and dangerous intrusion into our bodies is warranted, and perhaps even overdue. It is the basis of the growing interest in alternative medicines and treatments, holistic approaches, Eastern medical regimens, herbal remedies, and "New Age" medicine.

Generally speaking, there are two groups of women who seek natural solutions to their health questions: (1) Women who want to take nothing at all, who believe all supplemental medicine is somehow unnatural or chemical; and (2) Women who don't mind taking supplements, as long as those supplements are derived from natural substances.

And yet . . . we need to guard against throwing the proverbial baby out with the bathwater. It is all too easy to allow fear and cultural bias, fueled by our own bad experiences, to cause us to discard the brilliant and widespread improvements in our lives brought about by twentieth-century Western medicine. Aspirin, antibiotics, allergy drugs, and antidepressants are all widespread, acceptable, yet decidedly "non-natural" treatments that many people don't think twice about taking. Those same people balk at the mere mention of hormone replacement therapy. Many women who are reluctant to take estrogen are on tranquilizers and antidepressants, sleep medicines, pain medicines, and so on, all in an effort to suppress symptoms that would more effectively be treated with estrogen replacement. (One gets the feeling that if estrogen were also a diet pill, no one would question taking it, regardless of risk.)

In addition, the politicization of women's bodies that has taken place over the last few decades makes it difficult for any woman to exercise her choice independently and of her own free will. A woman whose symptoms are light enough to "go natural" may put pressure on a woman who has more severe symptoms to do the same thing. It is similar to the ongoing breast-feeding and natural-childbirth controversies that have been fought for some time now. Somehow, a woman who wants to take advantage of medical science to improve her own comfort, extend her life, and improve her health is "politically incorrect."

I hope the error of thinking exclusively that way is self-evident.

The question of what is "natural" and what is not is not always the right question to ask. Sometimes, one must ask what is healthy, what improves my life, and what makes sense. After all, cigarettes and alcohol might be considered "natural," but few people would actually consider them "good" for you.

Is it natural that the human life span is longer than it has ever been? Is it natural that rather than die shortly after their last child was born (as women in the long-ago past used to do), women today live as much as half of their lives after menopause? It seems far more *unnatural* that a woman lives half her life without vital hormones that are critical to her health and well-being.

In short, estrogen is not unnatural, and neither is estrogen therapy. Nor is the question either/or, black or white. Doctors and patients need to look at hormone replacement therapy not as a stand-alone treatment, but part of a whole-body/whole-life therapy, which might include antioxidants, vitamins, minerals, diet, and, if necessary, thyroid and other hormones that are lacking. The duration of hormone replacement therapy may be short term, long term, for life, or not at all.

Science has no proof that natural interventions are safer than synthetic. Despite the lack of proof, most of us perceive this as fact.

Natural hormones are those that occur in nature from either

plant or animal sources and are identical in chemical structure to the hormones occurring in the body. The plant sources that are usually available include soybean (estrogen) and wild yams (progesterone). All natural products may have allergic potential and may cross-react with each other, with the body's own chemistry, or with other substances. The unique problem of the allergic woman also needs to be considered, when choosing natural hormones.

Synthetic hormones are those that are produced in a lab. They may mimic hormones that are produced naturally in the body, and may even be chemically identical to natural hormones, but they do not occur in nature. The intention of synthetic hormones is generally to provide the same beneficial effects as natural ones, while being easier to produce, having fewer side effects, or being more specific to certain receptors in the body, and thus having a more localized effect.

Forms of Estrogen and Other Hormones

Both natural and synthetic hormone compounds can be placed in different "media" and utilized in many ways: injections, lotions, cream, gels, oral pills, sublingual pills, patches, and custom formulas. Much more widely available than in the past are "compounded" (custom-blended) hormones. With their more recent history we don't have a complete picture of their benefits and risks.

Natural hormones available for use in compounded formulas include:

- Estriol (E3 estrogen)
- Estradiol (E2 estrogen)
- Estrone (E1 estrogen)
- Progesterone
- Testosterone

They are prescribed in specific ways and can be filled only at special "compounding pharmacies" that prepare these products.

Some of the more common recipes produced are described by type of hormone. For example, estradiol gel is a water-based mixture of concentrated hormone and an inert gel that is rubbed into the abdomen or inner thigh. It is useful when women don't tolerate oral medication, or have trouble adjusting the dosage. The absorption may vary due to different skin types or varying techniques. If you need higher doses, it is better to order a concentrated gel with a higher concentration of estradiol, rather than using more gel at a lower concentration.

As their names would suggest, the biestrogens or triestrogens are blends of two or three types of estrogen.

- Biestrogen includes 20 percent estradiol (E2) and 80 percent estriol (E3).
- Triestrogen includes 10 percent estrone (E1), 10 percent estradiol (E2), and 80 percent estriol (E3).

Some women may get relief from symptoms by using these mixtures, yet find that the benefits are not always substantiated by a measurable change in their estrogen levels. Estrogen of different sources and formulas may interchange, but not all estrogens are well absorbed or provide desired effects and safety margins for every individual. A certain amount of trial and error is needed to find the proper balance. Diligent supervision will prevent risks and verify adequate protection.

Biestrogen and triestrogen may be taken orally in a number of different dosages. Transdermal or "patch" regimens that rely on direct absorption through the skin are available as well.

Estriol (E3) is the estrogen made by the placenta during pregnancy. It has been a source of renewed interest because there has been anecdotal data of the excretion of estriol in women with lower instances of breast cancer. Because of this, estriol has been described as potentially safer and causing less breast-cell stimulation than other forms of estrogen. However, it is still very likely to adversely stimulate the uterine lining if the dose and duration of therapy is equivalent in potency to the other estrogens, so it should be balanced by a progestin.

One downside of estriol is that it does not control symptoms well in many women. More research is needed to determine whether better outcomes relate to the type or dose of estrogen.

Non-estrogen alternatives that may be considered for treating hot flashes include Clonidine and Catapres (blood pressure medications) and Bellergal (a sedative/tranquilizer).

Testosterone

The "other" hormone we are all hearing about, the so-called miracle drug that restores our youthful sexuality and increases our sex drive . . . well, not exactly. The truth is sometimes it works, sometimes it doesn't. It can be a gel, cream, lozenge, or ointment. It can be used locally or taken in a method that distributes through the body.

Side effects may include acne, irritability or hostility, oily hair and skin, hair growth, and voice deepening. Careful monitoring is required so side effects can be detected early and avoided by decreasing the dose or eliminating it.

The testosterone lozenge is a soft, chewy, orange- or mint-flavored tablet that melts at warm temperatures. You dissolve a half lozenge in your mouth next to the cheek, approximately three times a week. If after two to three weeks there is no improvement, it can be increased to four times a week. If needed, after two to three weeks of four doses a week, the dosage can be adjusted upward to five times a week. This usually handles most women's loss of libido symptoms (if it's going to work) and dosage can be decreased over time to a maintenance level.

Testosterone ointments, gels, or creams are usually used directly on the vulva area once or twice a day. The amount also can be decreased over time when benefits are realized.

Progesterone Cream

The type and proper usage of the number of progesterone creams available varies widely; not all creams are alike. Many are not standardized or don't include pure or natural ingredients. Some don't contain any of the hormones claimed. The "placebo effect"—in which people respond positively to a substance with no active ingredients—is very powerful, making it difficult in some cases to determine whether the treatment is making a physical difference and if so, how much.

Progesterone is commonly available in 1.5 percent strength, and is used both for PMS (premenstrual syndrome) and as an adjunct to estrogen replacement. If it is used for PMS, it requires about 1 to 4 doses of 1 gram of 1.5 percent cream per day, over about 10 days prior to the onset of the period. This treatment is still considered controversial and has as many supporters as doubters. The variables that must be accounted for in PMS make it difficult to study and draw conclusions.

Progesterone cream replacement therapy protects the uterus, if about 1 gram of 10 percent cream is used twice daily. The lining of the uterus must be monitored for thickening (which is a precancerous potential, in which case biopsies are done), because absorption of the hormone and proper doses for protection vary. It is usually rubbed into the inner thigh, the underarm, or palms of the hand. Ultrasound measurement of the uterine lining can be an effective screening test to avoid an excessive number of biopsies; abnormal bleeding always requires a tissue sample.

Progestin can also be delivered to the system by the use of progesterone type IUDs (intrauterine devices), which also work as birth control. IUDs have their risks, but are a good choice in well-selected candidates. These are new IUDs, and are not associated with the dangerous side effects of IUDs reported in the past. They have a different structure and use new, safer materials.

Progestins can be delivered by injections, vaginal suppositories, oral pills, and "custom" (prescription) gels and creams as well. Remember, over-the-counter, nonprescription creams do not necessarily have enough progesterone, or indeed *any* of the type of progesterone needed to protect the uterus from cancerous change.

It is also possible to take progestins in combination with estrogen, via a transdermal (through-the-skin) patch called Combi-

Patch. You know those nicotine patches to help smokers quit cigarettes? Instead of nicotine, the CombiPatch delivers estrogen and
progesterone. The patch is a small, adhesive-backed circle that at-
taches to various locations on your body. (Unlike a nicotine patch,
it is not necessarily stuck to your upper arm.) It is great for women
who can't, won't, or don't remember to take pills.

Shop for prices on these items, as price will vary in some areas.
If you live far from the nearest compounding pharmacy (there are
many more than there used to be), mail order is readily available.
By the time you read this, it may even be possible to purchase hormones via the Internet, but please utilize these services with the
help of a professional.

It is important to keep in mind that many of the alternative and
natural regimens do not have clear safety and supervision guidelines available. Extra precautions and diligent follow-up with your
physician must be done to protect you from untoward side effects
and risks from newer, unproven regimens. This does not mean they
cannot be used relatively safely and effectively with the proper precautions, but you cannot assume they are low-risk or no-risk.

If you are dead-set on avoiding hormone replacement therapy,
it may be possible to reduce your symptoms in other ways, at least
for a while. Avoiding hot foods or drinks, alcohol, caffeine, and
warm environments may minimize hot flashes. Vitamin E may help
reduce them as well. Some herbs, such as dong quai, ginseng, and
black cohosh, are reputed to relieve flashes and other symptoms;
but for the most part, studies are inconclusive or negative. Fans
(ceiling, hand, or floor models) can help keep you cool, both to
reduce the likelihood of a flash and to help you feel more comfortable when you do get one. Layered clothing that may be easily removed and put back on may also help reduce some of the
discomfort when a flash occurs. Exercise may help with both osteoporosis and cardiovascular fitness, and calcium and vitamin D can
help bone strength. Vaginal moisturizers and lubricants can help
with dryness, while Kegel exercises may help reduce incontinence.

For women who don't mind taking other drugs and are just trying to avoid estrogen, bisphosphonates, calcitonin-salmon, and
raloxifene will help with osteoporosis, while Clonidine, Prozac (and

certain other antidepressants), and some natural progestins may help with other symptoms.

Finally, for those who are only trying to avoid oral estrogen, local and transdermal or subdermal estrogens may provide an alternative. Local estrogens include creams, gels, and the estrogen ring, Estring. Transdermal and subdermal estrogens include the estrogen patch and Norplant subdermal capsule.

If you are already on estrogen, and have decided to stop taking it, be sure to inform your health-care provider, so you can receive help doing it properly. It is important to taper off slowly, and not stop "cold turkey," or you may develop severe side effects. Don't let anyone intimidate you into sticking with a treatment you don't want. Nobody should be angry with you or refuse to care for you on the basis of your decision not to take estrogen.

Janice, the aerobics instructor at the beginning of this chapter, agreed to follow my advice to review a detailed journal of symptoms for four weeks. When she saw clearly how the severity and frequency of her symptoms were interfering with her daily life, we designed a custom-blended natural cream with estrogens and progesterones for daily use. We carefully adjusted the amount at four- to six-week intervals, settling on a blend of estradiol (E2) 0.5mg, estriol (E3) 2.0mg, and progesterone 50mg rubbed daily into the skin. This required a lot of appointments, but increased her chance of success. She is doing well now and we adjust her dosage as needed. We will reevaluate estrogen yearly, incorporating all the new information available. She may or may not choose to continue hormone replacement in the long term. This will be her decision as changing personal factors and new scientific information are revealed and, most of all, as her comfort level with the treatment is established.

The Gospel Truth—LIFE WITHOUT ESTROGEN: "I Prefer Aging the 'Natural' Way."

• • •

1. Your body needs estrogen to remain in its "natural" state. Going without estrogen is as unnatural as a diabetic going without insulin.

2. Although we have a greater concern now for unnecessary medication, and not unnecessarily tampering with our bodies' chemistry, we must be careful not to throw the baby out with the bathwater by denying our bodies essential, natural substances that it may no longer manufacture itself.

3. Many times, women take antidepressants, sleep medicines, pain medicine, and other drugs to mask or suppress symptoms more readily and effectively treated with estrogen.

4. Estrogen should not be viewed as a stand-alone treatment or cure-all, but as part of a whole-body health regimen that might include antioxidants, vitamins, minerals, diet, exercise, and other supplements as necessary.

5. Most of us perceive that natural interventions are safer than synthetic, even though there is no "proof" of this perception.

6. "Natural" does not always equate with "good." Cigarettes and alcohol may be considered natural, but they are not good for you. Furthermore, it is sometimes difficult to determine what is natural and what is not.

7. Estrogen is not unnatural, and neither is estrogen therapy.

7

TESTS
"My Doctor Did Blood Tests and They Are All Normal, So I Can't Be Menopausal."

● ● ●

Anita, a dentist in practice about 20 years, married with no children, told me:

"I've already seen my primary-care physician because I was concerned that I was starting the menopause. I'm 48 years old, and my periods still occur fairly regularly, although I miss one now and again. But I went to see him because I was very concerned about my memory. I was forgetting telephone numbers and addresses that I had committed to memory for many years. I find myself sitting in one place staring out into space and feeling like I'm in a fog. When I'm at work and need to concentrate, this is particularly distressing. At home I find myself walking into rooms and forgetting what I was going there for. I'm not having any hot flashes, but I usually wake up at about the same time every night, about 3:30 A.M., and I'm usually unable to get back to sleep for two or three hours. When I wake up in the middle of the night, my head starts spinning through all sort of negative life scenarios and I experience an overwhelming feeling of doom. Intellectually, I know that there's nothing terrible going on, but I still can't control the feeling. When my physician evaluated me, he ran a full battery of hormone tests, and he said they're all completely normal. I was so hoping there would be an abnormality and that the menopause might be responsible; but if the

lab tests were normal, I guess not. I'm here for a second opinion because I just know there's something not right. I know my own body."

Anita was right.

One of the typical effects of estrogen deficiency is waking up between 2 and 4 A.M. night after night, as Anita was. In fact, many parts of her story are classic complaints of hormone deficiency and are easily monitored for improvement.

Two hormone-level tests are commonly done to determine a woman's hormone level as it relates to menopause: FSH (follicle stimulating hormone) and estradiol (a type of estrogen commonly measured). FSH levels rise in the bloodstream as the ovaries lose their ability to respond and produce estrogen. The brain continues to produce FSH because it doesn't sense estrogen production, and the levels rise in a measurable amount. The ovaries' inability to produce estrogen lowers its levels in the blood and tissues, and over time estrogen levels steadily drop to become almost undetectable. The actual number that defines the menopause level varies from laboratory to laboratory: a common definition is an FSH level of about 25mIU/mL (25/1000 of an International Unit per milliliter) or more. Alternatively, if the FSH level is greater than 5mIU/mL on day three of the menstrual cycle, it also indicates low ovarian reserves.

In some cases, the FSH levels can remain in the normal range because *some* estrogen is being circulated—enough to manage the brain's production of FSH—even though the amount of estrogen is not enough for a particular individual to be entirely free of symptoms.

The estradiol level test is a more direct measure of estrogen in the blood, but it, too, can provide misleading results. The estrogen it detects may be present, but at the same time may be bound, inactive, or metabolized too rapidly, resulting in the menopausal symptoms. It is also subject to variation over the menstrual cycle and confusion due to foods, supplements, and other medications with estrogen and estrogen-like ingredients (such as certain wrinkle creams).

The problem is that neither of these tests is diagnostic. First of all, the timing of the tests influences their accuracy, because your hormone levels change over the course of the month. Particularly during menopause, estrogen levels can vary widely—from extreme highs to extreme lows—during the course of the month and even during a single day. Second, no one can say what your hormone levels "should" be, because each woman in the prime of her hormone-producing life has a different level of hormones. These tests give you a snapshot of your levels today, but say nothing about the more critical measure: how much hormonal *change* you are experiencing.

A woman and her doctor have to look beyond the lab tests. Determining appropriate levels is more a diagnosis of positivity than negativity. When FSH is too high, you've probably got estrogen deficiency, yet if the FSH measurement is normal, you still can't rule out estrogen deficiency. Normal estradiol readings also do not rule out estrogen deficiency. The readings obtained by these tests must be balanced against other symptoms a woman may be having and placed in their proper perspective.

That's why I am an advocate of what I call a "female thumbprint": At least once, before entering menopause, women should have their doctors measure the hormone levels that are appropriate for their bodies, assuming they're functioning well. The doctor can help determine the best timing for this, with regard to menstrual cycle, other medications, and variables that could affect the result. Later in life, diagnosis will be much simpler if the physician has a reference point of how the healthy, premenopausal patient measured on the standard tests.

The female thumbprint does not completely eliminate the unknowns from the equation, but it helps. Still there are questions that even this approach cannot answer. For example, does your tissue respond differently to hormone levels over time? The levels of hormones you produce at 35 may not be appropriate at age 50. Or, more worrisome, what if your natural level is higher than average, increasing your risk of breast cancer? Since hormone therapy may statistically increase the risk of breast cancer for some women, we obviously would not want to attempt to replicate your natural hormone levels in this case, because those levels may have been unsafe to begin with. We may in fact want to block these agents' activity at the receptors in the breasts to prevent breast cancer, by using special medicines that have that effect.

How did we solve our patient, Anita's, dilemma? She did not have a "thumbprint" I could work from. We started her on a cyclical oral regimen, allowing a withdrawal period to imitate her natural monthly cycle. We adjusted her doses several times in six months to eliminate bleeding between menstrual cycles. Her original progesterone dose was too high and caused some depression. Fifty percent of the original dose worked well; bleeding mid-cycle has stopped, and she's feeling herself again. The ultrasound revealed a thin uterine lining despite her lower dose of progesterone, a positive indication. Six months' evaluation initially and annual reevaluation to follow up will keep her on target as her body's hormones continue to change. Anita's treatment is a continual, dynamic process.

The Gospel Truth—TESTS: "My Doctor Did Blood Tests and They Are All Normal, So I Can't Be Menopausal."

• • •

1. There are two measurements commonly used to determine whether a woman is menopausal: the levels of FSH (follicle stimulating hormone) and estradiol in the blood. When FSH levels are high, estrogen is assumed to be low. Estradiol is a more direct measurement, but it may be misleading, because it can be detecting estrogen that is present, yet unavailable to the body. Neither test is accurate or necessary for diagnosis.

2. Timing may interfere with the results of hormone-level tests.

3. Women should consider taking a "female thumb-print," or baseline hormone-level test, before they are menopausal.

4. Listen to your body. If something doesn't feel right, it probably isn't, regardless of what tests say.

8

CANCER
"My Family History Makes Me Afraid to Take Estrogen."

● ● ●

Evelyn, a divorced 52-year-old woman with a strong family history of breast cancer and two daughters she's concerned about, told me:

"My mother died of breast cancer at 56. In those days, there wasn't a whole lot they did for the disease, nor were they detecting it early. I do know that she wasn't taking hormones. Nevertheless, as I find myself facing the estrogen decision, I am reluctant because of my mother's breast cancer. None of my sisters or aunts had it, but you never know; they might still develop it. Unfortunately, I have a history of osteoporosis and heart disease in my family as well. I need help to analyze my risk and possible benefits of hormone replacement therapy. Obviously, I don't want to take anything that would give me cancer."

I don't want to give Evelyn anything that will give her cancer either. And a family medical history is certainly a factor to take into consideration. Sometimes you grow up with family history; sometimes you don't find out what your family's medical background is until you're an adult, if at all. When it comes to cancer, any history at all is significant to us: Whether there is just one person in your family who has had cancer or several, it changes your perception.

But the fact is, women seem to get breast cancer regardless of their history: The largest percentage of women who get breast cancer have no family history of it at all. Furthermore, studies show that the rate of breast cancer recurrence correlates with the size of the original tumor, its stage, and its grade, not with being in a high-estrogen state, such as pregnancy.

In the U.S., it is reported that one woman in eight will get breast cancer in her lifetime. For heart disease, the risk is one in two. In terms of morbidity (death) rate, eight times as many women die of heart attacks than breast cancer. Estrogen therapy may increase the risk of breast cancer in some women, but it will decrease the risk of heart disease in almost all women.

So where is the balance?

Somewhere between healthy life, healthy heart, healthy bones, and breast-cancer risk, there's got to be a balance. To date, the most rigorous studies can't prove a relationship between short-term (less than 5 years) low-dose hormone replacement and in-creased breast cancer. The risks that researchers have documented are apparent only after 5–10 years of use. That does not explain the many cases of breast cancer in women who have never taken re-placement therapy—or the increase in breast cancer among younger, premenopausal women. It doesn't explain how estrogen therapy could be responsible for increased breast cancer when most women don't take estrogen replacement!

So much has been made in the media of the risk of breast can-cer for women taking estrogen that it discourages many people from even considering hormone replacement therapy. In fact, the possible link between hormone replacement therapy and breast cancer has been characterized as "the source of most of the con-troversy surrounding hormone use in postmenopausal women."[10] But is this logical? Breast cancer is common and will occur with great frequency in both estrogen users and non-users. It may not follow that it is cause and effect. Yes, there are some women whose personal medical background or family history warrants very seri-ous consideration of estrogen versus cancer risks; however, for the vast majority of women, the benefits far outweigh any risk of can-cer. The diseases that estrogen prevents are diseases that pose a *far* greater risk to most women than breast cancer, and it has been re-peatedly shown in study after study that the overall death rate, from all causes, for women on hormone replacement therapy is much lower than for those who are not. (This may be because of regular physician supervision during therapy.)

It should also be noted that early breast disease may be curable, while heart disease assuredly is not. Furthermore, heart attacks are more likely to be fatal in younger women. Recent statistics show that while younger men are likely to survive a first heart attack, younger women are less likely to. In contrast, the five-year survival rate for breast cancer is now as much as 95 to 97 percent.

What are the risk factors for breast cancer? They include the following, some well-described and acknowledged in the medical literature, others not yet proven:

- Family history
- Beginning periods before age 12
- Never having kids, or having first child after age 30
- Being more than 20 percent over your ideal weight
- Drinking more than 1½ glasses of wine daily
- Lack of exercise
- Having a diet low in vegetables and fruit and high in fat
- Exposure to high-dose radiation

Some feel that exposure to toxins, such as pesticides, is also a risk factor. More investigation is needed to determine the effect of these exposures.

Overall, if you don't take hormones, the risk of breast cancer is about 10 per 100 (regions will vary). If you take estrogen for 5 to 15 years, your risk is estimated at 13 to 14 per 100. An increase, but not a dramatic one.

All risk factors must be more fully examined to be fully understood: Even lack of family history is not necessarily an indicator of lower risk, as far more women with no family history at all are diagnosed with breast cancer than women with a family history. Still, when it comes to the "Big C," it is difficult to weigh statistics, balance risk factors, ignore emotions, and calmly decide that it's okay to take any risk at all. The fact is, while studies have shown a definite relationship between *estrogen levels* in a woman's body and breast cancer, they have not shown a definite link between *estrogen therapy* and breast cancer. Additional studies are needed to determine the risks, risk factors, and considerations a woman must keep in mind when considering hormone replacement therapy. We simply need to know *more!* What do we conclude of the 70 percent of all women with breast cancer who had no risk factors at all? What about causes such as viruses or bacteria? Crazy? They laughed about bacteria causing ulcers and guess what? It's true.

Breast Examination

• • •

A well-considered evaluation of your personal and family history, mammography, exercise, and diet, and regular self- and physician-examination should be a consistent part of the lifestyle of any woman over 40, regardless of whether or not you decide to take estrogen. All women should learn how to perform breast self-examination. It is an important line of defense against breast cancer, and done regularly once a month is one of the best tools available in early detection. Mammograms should be done at the interval recommended by your doctor (typically once every year or two after 40 and annually after 50), as it can detect a breast growth too small to be felt in self-examination. In fact, breast cancer can be detected by mammogram up to two years before a woman can detect it by self-examination, offering a major head start in treatment.

The key to the estrogen decision is balancing the risks and benefits on an individual, rather than a statistical, basis. For example, the fear of breast cancer may cause a woman to decide against estrogen based on the statistics, yet that decision may expose her to a higher risk of possibly fatal colorectal cancer, if there is a personal history of that in her family. If a woman has a family history of both breast and colorectal cancer, the decision becomes even tougher!

It may seem like one of those cruel medieval tortures, where inquisitors forced their victims to choose how they would die, but we hope that by carefully balancing the statistics with a woman's personal profile, we can remove most of the fear and horror of such a difficult decision.

Fifty thousand Americans die of colon and rectal cancer each year, more than half of them women. Colorectal cancers rank third in cancer incidence, behind lung and breast cancer. (Skin cancers are usually excluded from these statistics, because they are so common, and of so many types, they cannot be easily classified in this manner.)

Estrogen replacement therapy appears to reduce the risk of colorectal cancer by as much as 35 percent. This protection extends for several years after a woman stops the therapy, and then her risks return to the same rate as the general population.

Scientists currently believe that this benefit derives from the fact that estrogen reduces the production of secondary bile acid, which may be cancer-promoting. There has also been some evidence that estrogen may prevent cancer-cell growth. This fact alone is not a reason to use it, but it must be added to the equation.

Both breast-cancer screening by mammogram and cervical-cancer screening by Pap test are well known and accepted. You've probably read the good news that new cervical screening tests such as PapSure® have increased the accuracy of Pap tests from 60 to almost 90 percent. But the proper screening and evaluation of colon cancer is less well known and not widely discussed.

Compounding the issue is the uncomfortable nature of some testing, such as sigmoidoscopy, in which a telescope-like instrument is inserted through the rectum to view the lower gastrointestinal (GI) tract, or colonoscopy, in which the entire GI tract is viewed. Few of us stand in line to be first.

However, many experts believe routine screening via sigmoidoscopy or colonoscopy beginning at age 50 is a reasonable guideline. Testing for blood in the stool can be helpful as well, and is recommended yearly after about the age of 40. Don't ignore the possible warning signs, such as change in bowel habits, blood in stool, undiagnosed abdominal pain, or bloating.

Well-documented risk factors include a family history of polyp disease, history of other cancers, and some types of inflammatory bowel disease. Other suspected factors include high-fat, low-fiber diets, and low levels of physical activity. Preventive measures include exercise, folic acid, lower fat in the diet, and maintaining ideal body weight. Of course, these same measures benefit us in many other ways as well and reduce our risk of other ailments.

Although other types of cancer have not necessarily been correlated with estrogen use, I'd like to discuss them here, because it is interesting to note the potential risk factors that *are* currently known.

Cervical Cancer Risk Factors

- Sexual intercourse at an early age
- Multiple partners
- Male partners who had multiple partners
- Genital warts
- HIV positive
- Smoking

Ovarian Cancer Risk Factors

- Age, particularly for women without children
- Family history
- There is some possibility of a linkage between talcum powder and ovarian cancer, so it should not be used in the genital area.

Previous pregnancy, past use of birth-control pills, having your tubes tied (sterilization or tubal ligation), or ovary removal seem to lower your risk.

Uterine Cancer Risk Factors

- Being above ideal body weight
- Diabetes
- High blood pressure
- Gallbladder disease

- Anovulation (long periods of time without ovulating—essentially, not having a period—except during pregnancy)
- Using estrogen replacement without progestin

Skin Cancer Risk Factors

- Excessive sun exposure—all types (squamous cell or basal cell)
- Family history of melanoma
- Fair complexion (melanoma)
- Exposure to certain chemicals

For many cancers, common risk factors are family history, being above ideal weight, lack of exercise, poor nutrition, smoking or alcohol use, and exposure to other toxins. Aside from family history, which we cannot change, these are all areas we have the chance to control. We should take advantage of this knowledge to begin applying some moderation in our lives where due, and reduce our risk factors as early as we identify them.

So, if a woman has a family history of heart disease, Alzheimer's, colon cancer, or osteoporosis, the risks of which are reduced by replacement therapy, is that a clear indication she should take it? Nothing is that simple, unfortunately.

Balance. Individual assessment. Dynamic response. Flexibility.

We have to get away from abrupt, emotional responses to a choice like this. We have to weigh the side effects, family histories, background, previous treatment, and available choices that remain. Everything must be evaluated carefully and objectively, based on all the information at hand, and if additional information comes to light at a later date, then everything needs to be reevaluated and choices reconsidered. The individual nature of each woman must be paramount, and the physician or other provider should remember the need for flexibility in treatment, regardless of their interpretation of scientific facts.

Fortunately, the science and art of hormone therapy is advancing steadily. Replacement therapies will become more and more sophisticated, and additional choices will become available. It will become easier to administer more precise and more appropriate proportions of the right hormones, minimizing your exposure to risk factors and side effects, while maximizing the benefits. The "designer" estrogens, as they are called—new, synthetic estrogens that attempt to interact with certain parts of the body, but not with others—may provide specific benefits while eliminating other risks. It will take time to reach these goals, but we will. An example of designer estrogens, raloxifene, is already on the market: It targets specific receptors, avoiding breast and uterine receptor stimulation, while it prevents osteoporosis and improves the lipid profile.

These advances in hormone therapy come not only from improved medical understanding of the interrelation of the hormones and of their interaction with the body, but also from an improved pharmaceutical ability to prepare the needed compounds. Both custom titration, which is the ability to derive very precise amounts of a drug, and compounding, which is the ability to combine and manufacture a specific dose, are becoming ever more available. Large mail-order compounding pharmacies are increasing the availability of hormones in precise prescriptions to match a patient's physiological profile. Patients in rural or suburban areas now have access to treatments that were previously only available to women living in large cities.

Still, a major difficulty in obtaining good hormone therapy is that only a few doctors and practitioners are experienced, knowledgeable, and interested. Many others are experimenting without experience or sticking to a one-size-fits-all regimen. There can be a significant and frightening cost both to women and to the reputation of hormone treatment as a whole. DHEA is a good example. When certain unsubstantiated reports were released touting the hormone DHEA (dehydroepiandosterone) as a virtual "cure" for aging, it became the rage. A naturally occurring substance, and therefore not subject to FDA regulation, DHEA became available in health food stores and supermarkets, allowing people to self-prescribe large doses of the hormone. Yet all of the claims for the supposed effects of DHEA were hearsay, based on animal studies that had never been proven relevant to humans. Worse, some of these same studies showed that while DHEA had some positive effects on the rats being tested, it was also causing liver cancer. Even more dangerous, some people with the attitude of "If one is good, two must be better," were taking higher than recommended doses, with potentially toxic effects. How ironic that we are much more willing to take an unknown substance whose risks are undetermined than a more established substance with a longer safety record.

So while I don't think a woman should be *afraid* to take estrogen, regardless of her history, she should be *cautious,* as with any other therapy. It is important to interview your physician to determine her or his experience with hormone replacement therapy, views on the therapy and menopause in general, and understanding of the current state of the art of replacement, including its different approaches and applications.

We chose to start Evelyn, the woman who was concerned about breast cancer (in addition to her family history of heart disease and osteoporosis), on a new "designer estrogen" called raloxifene (brand name Evista®). This recently available compound can prevent osteoporosis and improve heart health, yet does not adversely stimulate the breast and uterus. It may even help protect the breast. Raloxifene does not relieve memory loss or hot flashes, but Evelyn didn't have these symptoms, so for her it was a perfect match. She will be followed with blood panels monitoring her heart health factors, such as cholesterol, triglycerides, and lipids. Calcium was added to her diet and strengthening exercises have been added to her daily exercise regimen. We will also do periodic bone-density evaluations and compare them to her baseline to assure the therapy is working. At 12 months, she is doing well. Her cholesterol is down to 200 from 250 and her bone density is stable. She tolerated the therapy with very few side effects.

The time that Evelyn remains on raloxifene will depend on its continued effectiveness and lack of side effects. Tamoxifen, a related substance, has shown promise as a preventative in women at high risk for breast cancer, and now raloxifene is being studied for this potential as well. Tamoxifen, unlike raloxifene, does stimulate the uterus and can cause precancerous and cancerous change. Women on tamoxifen for long periods as treatment or prevention need supervision to catch this problem early.

The Gospel Truth—CANCER: "My Family History Makes Me Afraid to Take Estrogen."

• • •

1. The largest percentage of women who get breast cancer have no history of it at all in their family.
2. Approximately one woman in eight to ten will get breast cancer, depending on the region of the country. One in two is at risk for heart disease.
3. The diseases that estrogen prevents pose a far greater risk to most women than breast cancer does. In fact, while the risk of getting breast cancer may be slightly higher in women who take estrogen, the risk of dying from it appears to be lower, possibly because of better care from regular physician supervision.
4. Based on our current knowledge, many cancers and other conditions are not affected by estrogen at all.

9

BONES
"I Exercise and Take Calcium, So Osteoporosis Is Not a Problem for Me."

• • •

Sally, a married, 47-year-old elementary-school teacher and mother of two, told me:

"None of my parents or grandparents, as far as I know, had osteoporosis; they all lived well into their 90s. I've always been a very active woman. I have played tennis several times a week for many years. I have plenty of calcium in my diet and I take calcium supplements. So I'm very upset, because I recently had a screening bone-density scan that shows I have the beginnings of bone loss. I don't think that's possible, because of my healthy lifestyle: I don't smoke or drink—I even avoid caffeine. Besides, no one in my family history has it. My relatives have never even broken a bone."

Osteoporosis affects about 25 million Americans—80 percent of them women. The annual direct cost of health care is at least $13.8 billion. Current trends indicate the occurrence of osteoporosis may double in the next 20 years.[11]

Osteoporosis is a medical condition in which your bones are breaking down faster than they are being replaced by new bone. This process may also be referred to as "bone loss." Osteopenia, the precursor to osteoporosis, is a thinning of the bone without the actual defects that eventually occur with osteoporosis. It can be detected and treated in order to prevent osteoporosis. Osteoporosis is responsible for the shrinking of our height as we grow older, sometimes by as much as several inches. It is what makes falls so serious for the elderly, and why calcium is so critical in our diet when we're younger. We all have seen the humps or stooped backs, and heard about the broken hips and crushed vertebrae.

However, a humped back and "old lady shape" are probably the least of your problems if you have osteoporosis: It is estimated that 1.5 million Americans experience osteoporosis-related fractures each year.[12] That's a lot of broken bones!

Eighty percent of broken hipbones are caused by osteoporosis. Twenty percent of women who have a hip fracture die, usually within a year, due to complications. That is one in five—a frightening number. As many as 25 to 33 percent must stay an extended period in a nursing home, and 50 percent of the rest will never return to normal living.

In other words, almost nobody survives such a fracture without serious effects for the rest of their lives.

Osteoporosis is a silent killer. Like hypertension, you will not feel it or see it until years after it starts. It creeps up on a body, weakening it slowly, little by little—so slowly, many people don't think of osteoporosis as the deadly disease it is. In fact, the bone loss can start as young as age 35, creeping and increasing as you age, and ramping up rapidly around your menopausal years. Osteoporosis gives no warning signs until you lose height, get a curve in your spine, suffer pain, or break something. The most common site of damage from osteoporosis is not the hip, as many people believe, but the vertebrae of the back. Crushed vertebrae and back pain are often signs of osteoporosis, and spinal-compression fractures are common results of this bone erosion. These symptoms may be noted for the first time on a routine x-ray, although the osteoporosis itself may not. If your mother or grandmother suffers from chronic back pain due to an osteoporotic spine, you know how critically important it is.

An estimated 25 percent of women over 60 have spinal-compression fractures. These fractures ultimately lead to a loss of height, and if left untreated, could cost you as much as three inches in stature.

People often assume that because osteoporosis is silent, that it is also slow. It is slow to come to attention, but it is not slow in its changes. In fact, postmenopausal bone loss from osteoporosis averages 1 percent per year. For a woman of 75 who started menopause at 50, this means she may have lost as much as a quarter—25 percent—of her bone mass already!

Osteoporosis causes the mass of the bone to decrease, but it also disturbs the way bones are put together. Imagine a mason putting bricks down, making line after line into a straight wall, suddenly twisting the bricks together in different directions, leaving a brick out here and there, or using bricks made out of material that dissolves in water. Instead of a strong, straight wall, you end up with a disrupted structure with missing pieces that is susceptible to falling apart just from nature's elements or minimal trauma.

In the same way, osteoporosis doesn't just make a bone weaker but changes its structure in such a way that it affects its relationship to the other bones. This is another reason the bones are more susceptible to breaking.

Any time you break a bone due to low-impact trauma, especially if you are over 40, you should be suspicious of osteoporosis. But screening is important for everyone, because even if you are absolutely sure you don't have osteoporosis, like Sally, you just might anyway: There is no way to tell without specific osteoporosis testing. Most people think you can tell if you have osteoporosis, by a standard x-ray. You can't. The changes won't appear on a standard x-ray until almost half the bone is lost!

Fortunately, it has become relatively easy to detect osteoporosis and osteopenia. While in the past, many physicians didn't check for bone loss until a patient had suffered a break or injury, today it is possible to screen for bone loss as a part of a patient's regularly scheduled checkup.

There are two basic bone-screening processes: One is *central,* which takes measurements of the hip and spine as you lie on a special moving bed; the other is *peripheral,* which measures the forearm, the heel, or even the finger. Both feed the measurements into a computer, which compares them to those of a "control woman" with young, healthy bone.

The two most-common methods for each of these processes

have tongue-twisting names: dual-energy x-ray absorptiometry (DEXA) and quantitative computed tomography (QCT). Of the two, DEXA is the preferred method, and can be done in less than five minutes. It should be noted that DEXA only delivers about 10 percent of the radiation of a standard chest x-ray.

QCT is more expensive than DEXA and delivers a larger radiation dose, but may still be done in some facilities.[13] The machines used for DEXA are also very expensive, and may not be available at your doctor's health facility.

Other less-common methods have the equally tongue-twisting names of dual photon absorptiometry (DPA) and ultrasound transmission velocity, the latest method being evaluated.

For screening, both methods—central and peripheral—are useful, but central is more effective in monitoring ongoing treatment, namely, to see if what you are taking is working (as opposed to simply taking a one-time or occasional measurement).

In any case, the process is simple and noninvasive. The report it generates will give you a score for absolute bone mass (Z-score), bone mass relative to sex and age, and bone mass relative to the young adult mean (T-score).

You can use your T-score to figure out where you lie in the risk profile. It is generally accepted that:

- Young, normal bones have a T-score of -1.0 and above ("above" meaning less negative, e.g., scores such as -0.5 and -0.2)
- Osteopenia means the T-score is between -1.0 and -2.5. These bones are thinner, but without the defects and more extensive changes of osteoporosis.
- A T-score of -2.5 or lower (such as -2.7 or -3.0) indicates possible osteoporosis.

Unfortunately, these statistics and scores are based only on Caucasian women; more research is needed that is specific to heredity.

Whom should we screen and when should they have the screening done? According to the National Osteoporosis Foundation, women who have risk factors such as a:

- Family history of osteoporosis
- Personal history of low-trauma fracture after age 40–45
- History of smoking
- Thin frame with low body weight

should be screened at least once between the ages of 45 and 50. Additionally, women in the following groups should consider screening as well:

- Anybody with health issues known to increase osteoporosis, such as chronic steroid use, overactive parathyroid glands, hyperthyroidism, and thyroid medications.
- Women who are on the fence about hormone therapy or other therapies for bone loss.
- Women who have been on estrogen therapy for a few years, to make sure the expected protection is occurring. Not all women follow the graphs.

By their early 60s all women should have had at least one bone density evaluation to help plan future intervention in time to make a difference.

While the loss of estrogen in a woman's body has been shown to be the leading factor in the progression of osteoporosis (and the primary reason it affects women so much more than men), there are many other factors that can increase the risk. The consumption of cigarettes, alcohol, caffeine, and steroids, and hypothyroidism (low thyroid hormone levels), are some of the controllable factors that may increase a woman's chances of suffering from osteoporosis. Being thin or having a small frame can also increase your risk. A 50-year-old white woman is at 40 percent risk that she will experience either a vertebral, wrist, or hip fracture during the remainder of her life.[14] Some ethnic groups are more likely to experience osteoporosis, as are asthmatics and people taking steroid therapy. The National Osteoporosis Risk Assessment initiative (N.O.R.A.) recently conducted studies that indicate Hispanic, Asian, and Native American women may be at greater risk than Caucasian women for osteoporosis, while African-American women may be at lower risk.[15]

Estrogen preserves and may actually increase bone density with continued use. It greatly slows, halts, and sometimes even reverses the effects of osteoporosis and osteopenia, by helping the kidneys to reabsorb the calcium available in the bloodstream (instead of losing it in the urine), and slowing the dissolution of the bones. Estrogen use can decrease the risk of fractures related to osteoporosis by 50 to 60 percent. Combining estrogen with calcium reduces the risk of fractures as much as 80 percent. Estrogen therapy works best for osteoporosis if started early and maintained at least 8 to 10 years. But it's never too late; it helps prevent loss of bone density whenever you start.

Suggested doses of estrogen to treat and prevent osteoporosis vary, depending upon the estrogen supplement being used. While health professionals have long relied upon 0.625mg of Premarin or its equivalent daily, newer studies of some replacements, such as Estrace, show they are effective in as little as half the equivalent dose.

In addition to hormones, bone health depends on adequate calcium, vitamin D, and exercise. But while a diet rich in calcium, vitamins, and certain essential minerals will forestall or reduce osteoporosis, unfortunately it may not eliminate the risk entirely or significantly. Premenopausal women should take 1,000mg of calcium a day. After menopause, this may be increased to 1,500mg daily for women on estrogen, or 1,800mg to 2,000mg for women not taking estrogen. If possible, these doses should be achieved through a combination of diet (eating foods high in calcium) and supplementation. It is important to find a supplement with a high level of "elemental calcium," or calcium in its chemically pure form. Typically, supplements with calcium carbonate have the highest elemental calcium, but some people have stomach problems with calcium carbonate, and must try other forms such as lactate, citrate, or gluconate. These forms of calcium have as little as one-quarter the elemental calcium of calcium carbonate.

It should be noted that calcium supplements are absorbed better by your body when taken with food, and that splitting the dose by taking half the dose twice a day is better than taking the full dose once a day. Taking one-third of the dose with every meal would be great. Spreading the dose improves your body's ability to absorb the calcium and reduces any potential for gastric upset.

You need vitamin D to enhance the absorption of calcium. You can get it through sunlight or by supplementing with 200 to 400 IU (International Units) daily. Vitamin D intake of as much as 600 to 800 IU is recommended to reduce risk of fracture in older women who are primarily indoors. Unfortunately, sunscreen, which is very important to preventing skin cancer, does interfere with vitamin D absorption, but you only need 15 minutes of sun a day to get your recommended daily amount. Even fair-skinned people can usually get their full dose without skin damage. Vitamin D may be toxic in large doses, so avoid taking more than the recommended daily allowance.

Many people wonder about adding fluoride to their diets. Fluoride has proved helpful for strong teeth, but it doesn't seem to work the same way for bones. In addition to having side effects when taken in the amount necessary to strengthen bones, fluoride also does not seem to build good bone material—it builds quantity, but not quality. (Speaking of teeth, estrogen deficiency has been linked to accelerated tooth loss, so taking estrogen may help both your bones and your teeth.)

Exercise for your bones is defined as 30 to 40 minutes of weight-bearing activity, such as walking, at least three times a week. Use one- to-two-pound weights when you are doing your exercise, to build bone strength in the upper body as well.

Risk Factors for Osteoporosis

• • •

- Being white or Asian
- Alcohol
- Cigarette smoking
- Caffeine
- Animal protein (eating meat)
- Inadequate nutrition, especially lack of calcium
- Little or no physical activity
- Heredity

- Medications, most commonly steroids and thyroid hormone
- Loss of menstrual period for long intervals when you're younger, (i.e., extreme athletes and anorexic women or adolescents)
- Acidic foods, including colas and soft drinks
- Foods that are high in phosphorous, such as certain meat, fish, and cereals (which may bind the calcium in your body and prevent its absorption, when eaten to excess)

Like Sally, you may have thought that if you followed "the rules," by exercising and taking calcium, you couldn't get osteoporosis. Indeed, many people believe osteoporosis can only be helped by exercise and calcium. But while exercise and calcium can slow and reduce the effects of the disease, estrogen and other medications, such as Fosamax®, have been shown to slow, stop, and possibly even reverse the effects of osteoporosis—actually increasing your bone density. As screenings for bone-loss ratio have become more effective, women have a better opportunity than ever before to detect and prevent the effects of osteoporosis by initiating treatment early.

As we've noted, estrogen can reduce the risk of fractures due to osteoporosis by 50 to 60 percent. On the other hand, you should be aware that the benefits of estrogen do not remain after therapy is discontinued: Women who stop estrogen replacement will gradually lose its protection against osteoporosis, even if they've taken it for years.

Estrogen/androgen combinations can also help to decrease the resorption of bone, and potentially may help build it. Various non-estrogen treatments are available to women who can't take estrogen, but their benefits are restricted from the full array that estrogen may provide. Doctors may choose to prescribe non-hormone alternative treatments for osteoporosis for women with a strong family history of breast cancer, as well as other medical problems where hormones are contraindicated, such as severe liver disease. (As with many medications, estrogen is processed in the body by the liver.)

ESTROGEN ALTERNATIVES FOR OSTEOPOROSIS

Bisphosphonates

The bisphosphonates are non-hormone agents that prevent loss of bone. They are specific to bone and don't offer either the benefits or risks of estrogen in other organ systems.

Alendronate (brand name Fosamax®) is a type of bisphosphonate, and is the first treatment of its kind to be approved by the FDA for treating and preventing osteoporosis. While Fosamax has been touted in the media as an "alternative" to estrogen, it is only so for the prevention and treatment of osteoporosis, and not other menopausal symptoms. For example, Fosamax has not been shown to help with cardiovascular health, Alzheimer's disease, hot flashes, or incontinence. Additionally, it has its own set of rules and side effects with regard to dosage.

For example, Fosamax can wreak havoc on the stomach, and must be taken in a prescribed manner. A full 8-ounce glass of water must follow its ingestion on an empty stomach. To avoid damage to your esophagus, you must remain upright for at least 30 minutes after taking it. You also may not eat, drink, or take any other medication for a half hour after taking Fosamax.

A daily 5mg is the preventative dose and 10mg daily is the treatment dose. If all of the precautions are followed, treatment is likely to be "uneventful."

As with estrogen, women who stop taking Fosamax lose the benefits of its treatment soon afterward.

Other bisphosphonates are currently being investigated but have not yet received FDA approval for treating osteoporosis.

Calcitonin-salmon

Additionally, the FDA (federal Food and Drug Administration) has approved calcitonin-salmon (brand name Miacalcin®) as an osteoporosis treatment. Its efficiency in restoring bone density and reducing fractures is still under study. It may be administered as a nasal spray, and is recommended for women who are more than five years past menopause and cannot tolerate estrogen, refuse to take estrogen, or cannot take estrogen because of cancer risk or other problems. Women who take calcitonin-salmon are also advised to take calcium and vitamin D supplements, as well as to exercise regularly.

Calcitonin-salmon is well tolerated, safe, and has the interesting side benefit of helping with pain in women who already have osteoporosis.

Raloxifene

Raloxifene, a "designer estrogen" (brand name Evista®), has been FDA-approved for osteoporosis prevention. It belongs to the class of treatments called selective estrogen receptor modulators (SERMs). These are substances that selectively affect the estrogen receptors in your body, so, for example, the receptors that increase your bone density are stimulated, but the receptors that stimulate your breast tissue are not. A recent study indicates that two years of treatment with raloxifene may decrease the risk of certain fractures of the vertebrae by as much as 50 percent—about the same effect as estrogen.

Raloxifene is designed to have positive effects on bones and lipids but apparently does not increase stimulation of endometrial or breast tissues. This means little or no breast tenderness, and no bleeding problems or uterine cancer risk.

Raloxifene may not be as beneficial as either estrogen replacement therapy or Fosamax for preventing osteoporosis, but since it does not seem to increase the risk of breast or endometrial cancer, it may be a suitable alternative to estrogen. Its effects on fractures and cardiovascular health are still being studied.

Tamoxifen

Tamoxifen (brand name Nolvadex®) was the first SERM to be released, and has been used as a chemotherapy treatment for breast cancer, and in breast-cancer prevention trials. It appears to have an antiestrogen effect on breast tissue, and an estrogen-like effect on bones. It also stimulates the lining of the uterus, and has the potential risk of increasing uterine precancerous and cancerous changes.

TREATMENT VERSUS PREVENTION

Note that although osteoporosis can be *treated* with these various regimens, it can only be *prevented* by estrogen therapy, raloxifene (Evista), or alendronate (Fosamax), in combination with calcium and exercise.

How do we decide whom we should treat?

* If you've already broken your back or your hip, it is safe to say you have osteoporosis and should be treated.
* Any woman who has a T-score of -2 or lower.
* Any woman who has a T-score of -1.5, plus any of the other risk factors we have discussed, such as family history of osteoporosis, low-trauma fracture at a young age, history of smoking, thin frame with low body weight, etc.

Although it is never too late to start treating a woman for osteoporosis, the most rapid bone loss occurs in the first menopausal years, so preventative therapy during this time is the most effective. As we've mentioned before, the therapy is maintenance, not a cure, so if you discontinue it, you start losing bone again; within about four years or so, you will be back to where you started.

In addition to the prevention and reversal of the disease of osteoporosis itself through estrogen, calcium, and exercise, take action to reduce your risk of fractures in general:

* Avoid certain sedatives.
* Have your eyes checked.
* Eliminate things from your home that may cause you to slip or fall.
* If you need to reach something on a high shelf, use a

sturdy step stool or ladder, instead of a chair or ottoman.

- Never stand on anything that has wheels, unless it is designed for that purpose and the wheels can be locked.
- Remove loose rugs and correct or clearly mark uneven floor surfaces.
- If your home has stairs, keep them clean, be sure that they are not loose, or do not have a loose covering, and be sure they are lit.
- Don't wear high-heeled shoes. Even if you have strong legs or ankles, heels can break and soles may slip. If you are old enough to be at risk for osteoporosis, you are old enough to break a hip. Given the risks of permanent damage—or even death—from hip injury, high heels present an unreasonable risk. (Shoes with laces may also present a problem, especially if you have trouble tying them because of arthritis or eyesight problems.)
- If you have been diagnosed with osteoporosis, avoid things such as cycling, skiing, sky diving, and other activities with increased exposure to risk for falling unless treatment has brought your T-score into acceptable limits.

In one recent study, patients who were given guidance on how to avoid falls reduced their rate of falls and subsequent injury. The number of patients who reported any falls in a one-year period was 42 percent, compared to 68 percent in a group that was not given guidance. The number of patients reporting more than three falls was reduced by one-half. Serious fall-related injuries were reduced to 6 percent for the instructed group, from 10 percent for the uninstructed group, and hospital admissions were 69, compared to 97.[16]

We have some answers to osteoporosis, but at the same time, we have many more questions. Research continues and is needed to develop more SERMS (selective estrogen receptive modulators), new bisphosphonates that have fewer stomach side effects, and other new and exciting treatments that can prevent loss of bone and create new, healthy bone with little or no risk.

We started Sally on Fosamax, since she chose to avoid estrogen for the time being. We evaluated her exercise regimen and added weight training for her upper body, as well as 1,000mg of calcium as a supplement. Twenty-four months later we have repeated her scan and found the bone loss continuing, although at a much slower rate, and she has decided to begin low-dose estrogen therapy. Her bone density will be reevaluated at regular intervals and the treatment regimen augmented as appropriate.

The Gospel Truth—BONES: "I Exercise and Take Calcium, So Osteoporosis Is Not a Problem for Me."

• • •

1. Osteoporosis is a decrease in bone density that makes bones more brittle and easily breakable.
2. Osteopenia is a precursor to osteoporosis. It is defined as a thinning of the bone mass, without actual progression to osteoporosis.
3. Osteoporosis and osteopenia can be diminished by calcium in the diet and exercise, but estrogen is a much more potent prevention.
4. Most people associate osteoporosis with broken hips in the elderly, but the most common sites of fracture are crushed vertebrae.
5. Osteoporosis can be fatal: Complications caused by infections and other recovery complications associated with broken bones can actually kill.
6. So-called designer drugs like raloxifene and other medications, such as Fosamax, may be helpful in fighting osteoporosis, but may not help with other symptoms of menopause.
7. Your ethnicity and genetic predisposition may determine your susceptibility to osteoporosis, regardless of your health habits.

10

THE HEART
"I'd Rather Have a Heart Attack Than Get Breast Cancer."

• • •

Suzanne, a 51-year-old journalist, came to me with some concern.

She said *"It's been over a year since I had my last period. I've had all the classic menopausal and perimenopausal symptoms: hot flashes, night sweats, forgetful episodes. I've totally lost my sex drive; thank God I'm not involved right now. I look in the mirror and constantly imagine I'm getting a hump, like my mother, and I'm starting to get a little shorter, too. My regular doctor prescribed estrogen, but I didn't want to take it. He just shoved them across the desk, and said, 'They won't kill you!' My grandmother's sister had breast cancer, so although it's somewhat removed, I am concerned about my own risk of breast cancer and maybe it will kill me! I've read about estrogen decreasing the risk of heart disease. But breast cancer is so much worse—I think I'd rather have a heart attack."*

Suzanne is not atypical of women who come into my office: These are women who are well informed and, in some cases, more current on the latest fads than their physicians. These are women who are knowledgeable, yet fearful. A little knowledge is a dangerous thing.

Complete the following sentence: The number one killer of women is _____.

Many of you will say breast cancer, but you would be wrong. The answer is heart disease. (Breast cancer isn't even second. It now trails lung cancer as a cause of mortality in women.) The prevalence of death and disability due to heart disease in women has long been overlooked and underestimated. *The number of women in the U.S. who will die from some form of cardiovascular disease is more than double the number who will die from all forms of cancer combined.* Over 60 percent of women who die from cardiovascular disease had no previous symptoms, and 80 percent of the deaths due to cardiovascular disease in women under the age of 65 occur during their first cardiovascular "event." These women don't get a second chance.

Women often fail to have the "traditional" symptoms that men so commonly have, such as crushing chest pain going into the left arm. Rather, women may show very subtle signs, such as persistent tiredness, shortness of breath, or jaw discomfort. Women are often ignored when they complain of a problem, and the symptoms are confused with other more benign conditions. They then suffer another episode, often a more drastic event.

Although the number of studies is increasing, research in many areas of health is scarce for women, and is especially lacking in the area of heart disease. Breast cancer, while frightening and potentially devastating, is still curable in many cases. Heart muscle damage, however, particularly after an "event" (such as a heart attack), is not curable or even reversible.

In order to decrease the incidence of heart disease in women, we need a combination of:

- prevention
- early diagnosis
- effective treatment
- diligent follow-up

PREVENTION

Prevention efforts should focus on nutritional guidelines, exercise, family-history analysis, screening, and reducing risk factors. Risk factors for cardiovascular disease include:

- High blood pressure (above 130/80)
- Diabetes

- Aging
- Losing estrogen early (such as due to surgery, disease, or early menopause of any type)
- Smoking
- Hereditary factors, including high lipids (fat cells), premature heart events in the family (before age 60 in a mother or sister, before age 50 in a father or brother), and race
- High cholesterol and/or triglycerides
- Stress

Reducing your risk of heart disease before it happens can be achieved by trying to reach the following measurable goals:

Risk Factor	Measurement
Blood pressure	130/85 or less
LDL (low-density lipoproteins or "bad" cholesterol)	130mg/dl or less
HDL (high-density lipoproteins or "good" cholesterol	45mg/dl or more
Total cholesterol	200mg/dl or less
Triglycerides	200mg/dl or less

I cannot overemphasize the importance of diet in cardiovascular health, especially with regard to cholesterol, fat, lipids, and triglycerides. High levels of LDL ("bad cholesterol") and low levels of HDL ("good cholesterol") seem to be important factors in increased cardiovascular risk. The relevance of high triglyceride levels is still being studied, but they do seem to increase the risk of cardiovascular disease when a woman also has low levels of good cholesterol. You will improve your cholesterol profile by decreasing the amount of fat in your diet; eating less red meat and fewer fatty dairy products, and increasing the amount of lean poultry and fish and low-fat or nonfat dairy. Eating more vegetables, high-fiber foods, and grains seems to help the good-bad cholesterol balance, but actually may be due to less fat and fewer calories.

Exercise may be of even greater importance than diet. Getting at least 20 minutes of exercise three times a week that raises your pulse to optimum levels is critical to the health of your heart. (Longer intervals are needed for weight loss.) To determine your target heart rate, subtract your age from 220, and multiply the result by 75 percent. This is the ideal pulse rate you should reach and maintain for at least 20 minutes of cardiovasular exercise.

For example, if you are 50, your optimum pulse is: 220-50 = 170 x .75 = 127.5, or about 128 beats per minute (or 32 beats in 15 seconds).

Note that exercise for cardiovascular health is different in intensity and duration from the exercise you need to do if you are trying to lose weight or prevent osteoporosis. Fat burning usually requires 45 to 60 minutes of exercise, as often as five to six days a week, while exercise for your bones means 30 to 40 minutes at a time of weight-bearing exercise with resistance work. Regardless of what you hope to achieve, you should begin any new exercise program slowly, cautiously, and under a doctor's care. Get a checkup before you start.

Walking may be in many ways the easiest, safest, and most reliable workout for those who are new to exercise, or those who scoff at or can't afford health clubs, lycra, spandex and sweat. Start with 20 minutes, three times a week—perhaps only 10 minutes if you are very obese or completely out of shape. Gradually increase the distance, time, and pace of your strolls. A woman in her 50s or 60s should walk at a pace of about 3 miles per hour to reach her ideal pulse rate. The nice thing about walking is that it is practical. If you walk alone, you can use the time to think. If you walk with company, you can talk to your walking partner. You can walk to the store or post office and run an errand. If the weather is bad, you can walk around the mall; in fact, many malls offer walking programs for women, especially seniors, early in the morning. If you are so inclined, you can even use a treadmill at home, eliminating the need to leave the house altogether if the neighborhood is not so good for walking or the weather is too often wet.

Other forms of exercise, such as running, cycling, swimming, aerobics, and yoga, are also worth considering if you are physically capable. They all require specialized equipment or facilities and reasonably good physical health to begin with. To some extent, they also entail some degree of additional risk and are higher impact. This may cause long-term chronic injuries. However, if you enjoy these types of exercise, and possess the health to pursue them, they are beneficial. Remember always to warm up first, then stretch, then exercise, and finish with a cool down.

EARLY DIAGNOSIS

Early diagnosis will require better tests that predict problems prior to an "event" reliably and with cost effectiveness. Health-care providers may need to be reeducated to assess women more aggressively and evaluate symptoms early. Advancements in treatment itself are needed to bolster early intervention and improve access for women to the right kind of care.

EFFECTIVE TREATMENT

Estrogen relaxes the blood vessels, reducing blood pressure; it also lowers the low-density lipoproteins (LDL, or so-called bad cholesterol) that cause plaque in the arteries, and boosts high-density lipoproteins (HDL, or so-called good cholesterol). By narrowing the blood vessels, plaque robs the heart of oxygen and can actually increase blood-clot formation. It is very clear that estrogen lowers a woman's potential risk for cardiovascular disease, even if the mechanisms of *how* it works are unclear.

The new selective estrogen receptor modulators, called SERMs, have also shown promise in preliminary studies of reducing the risk of cardiovascular disease. These drugs, which include tamoxifen (brand name Nolvadex®) and the "designer estrogen" raloxifene (brand name Evista®), may be alternatives to "regular" estrogen for women who can't or won't take it. It is important to keep in mind that these drugs have their own risk profiles and side effects, making them a poor risk for some. Additional study is required to determine their efficacy in reducing cardiovascular risks over longer periods of time.

DILIGENT FOLLOW-UP

Once a woman has had a single cardiovascular event and survived it, follow-up with her physician needs to be very aggressive and persistent, in order to lower the risk of a second cardiovascular event. Better cardiac rehabilitation with a focus on health issues specific to women enhances the success of these programs by improving compliance.

Heart disease is largely preventable by reducing your risk factors. Tobacco is the worst offender, increasing risk of heart disease by at least 3 to 4 times the baseline. Cholesterol that is elevated, particularly the "bad" cholesterol, increases the risk of heart problems. A low-fat diet, exercise, cholesterol-lowering drugs, blood pressure medication, and hormone therapy can play a protective role. High blood pressure can also be reduced by exercise and the right kind of diet, which also may prevent or improve Type 2 diabetes, another risk factor in heart disease.

Diabetes and Estrogen

• • •

Diabetes, another ailment with no cure, affects 15 to 20 million people in the U.S. alone. It is a leading cause of death and disability. Half of the cases of diabetes in the U.S. occur in women over the age of 55—which makes the menopause a good time to test for it.

There are two types of diabetes: Type 1, in which the pancreas fails to make insulin, a hormone that helps the body regulate the metabolism of sugar; and Type 2, in which insulin is produced but is not effective in using sugar in the blood. Both types result in increased blood sugar.

Type 1 diabetes is hereditary, and requires insulin injections to maintain health. Type 2 diabetes can often be managed by weight loss, diet, exercise, and oral medication. Sometimes it, too, requires insulin. Type 2 diabetes is more likely if you are over 45 years old, have a positive family history, or are 20 percent or more over your target body weight. If you are inactive, test low for high-density lipoproteins (HDL, or "good" cholesterol), high for triglycerides, and high for blood pressure, you are also at increased risk.

Why are we talking about diabetes in the "heart" chapter? Because diabetes does not come alone. It can cause heart disease, as well as eye problems, nerve damage, and other serious problems. Signs and symptoms of possible diabetes include increased thirst, increased urination, increased fatigue, recurrent vaginal infections, and problems with nerves or vision.

If you have diabetes, you should be screened for heart disease, and you should aim for lipid and blood pressure levels that are more conservative than other people. It is not easy to do, but the investment in change is worth it.

We tested Suzanne for heart-disease factors, lipid profiles, and triglycerides, and took a careful family history. She did have increased triglycerides and cholesterol. I prescribed low-dose natural estradiol and placed her on a low-fat diet, monitored her for improvement in lipids, and suggested regular mammograms, breast exams, and semiannual visits. She also required progesterone, which I prescribed simultaneously with the estradiol, because she still has a uterus to protect. After 24 months, Suzanne is doing great. Her HDL lipids are up and her triglycerides are down. We continue to evaluate her health and progress on a semiannual basis.

The Gospel Truth—THE HEART: "I'd Rather Have a Heart Attack Than Get Breast Cancer."

• • •

1. Heart disease is the number one killer of women. In fact, a woman's first heart attack is more often fatal than a man's.
2. More medical research is necessary to bring women's cardiovascular care to parity with men's.
3. Heart disease is not curable, but it may be preventable.
4. The signs of heart disease in women may be much subtler than in men. Small signs may indicate significant disease and should be acted upon.

5. Diabetes can play a role in heart disease and other problems. Hormones can play a positive role in controlling blood-sugar levels and the incidence of Type 2 diabetes.

THE BRAIN
"I'm Having More and More 'Senior Moments.' Could I Be Getting Alzheimer's?"

• • •

Sylvia, a 52-year-old physician, came into my office visibly frightened and explained:

"I am living a nightmare," she said. "I can't remember phone numbers or people's names. One day recently, I was driving, and I didn't know how I got where I was. This really scared me. My mother has Alzheimer's, and I'm afraid I have it too!"

Almost everybody associates memory loss with aging. The term "senior moment" has crept into the popular vocabulary to describe those particularly vexing moments when we walk into a room, only to forget why, or when we spend a few minutes looking for the keys or glasses we clutch in our anxious hands. Even while we're still in our 20s, it is not uncommon to attribute those little memory hiccups of daily life to getting older. I find it amusing when a patient in her 40s attributes a moment of forgetfulness to "growing old." For most people, the effect of aging on the brain begins much older than that!

Yet beneath the quips and offhand remarks about "losing it" lie some very real fears about the true meaning of memory loss—the gradual slipping away into feebleness, senility, and even dementia. Severe, chronic memory loss is one of our most persistent fears when it comes to aging, characterized most strongly by our concern about being diagnosed with Alzheimer's disease.

Alzheimer's disease is a progressive disease of aging that affects one's *cognitive ability*—the ability to think, reason, and remember clearly. The earliest, most obvious, and best-known symptom is loss of memory. Short-term memory is usually affected first; Alzheimer's sufferers may find they can remember events of long ago, but not those from a few moments past. Additionally, they may find it difficult to perform complex tasks or remember a particular word; they may become disoriented.

These symptoms get worse as the disease progresses. Even simple tasks become difficult and speech may become incoherent. A variety of other symptoms may occur, from irritability and depression all the way to hallucinations and delusions. Alzheimer's patients may become disoriented in time and place; they may find it difficult to sleep, or to hold their bladders. In its worst stages, the disease may leave its victims entirely unable to care for themselves.

There are other senile dementias that are quite similar to Alzheimer's, so much so that a proper diagnosis can be tricky. Unfortunately, these other dementias may be no more treatable than Alzheimer's.

It has been estimated that nearly 50 percent of people over the age of 85 may be afflicted to some degree with Alzheimer's or other dementias.

Normal brain function depends upon many things. If you have ever been irritable from PMS, it won't be news to you that hormones affect your thoughts, attitudes, and capabilities, but it is only in recent years that scientists have begun to assess and quantify hormonal influences.

Ever find yourself in a room and not know how you got there? Ever have trouble remembering your own phone number? Ever put refrigerator items into an unrefrigerated kitchen cabinet? These are just a few examples of what your brain may do without estrogen.

Estrogen affects the health of the brain and central nervous system. It has been shown to improve mental health, elevating mood, improving cognitive ability (memory), and reducing the risk of dementia. It has been shown to increase blood flow in the brain, lowering the risk of both Alzheimer's disease and stroke. Estrogen may even increase the speed with which the brain processes information, decreasing reaction lag time and allowing women to respond more quickly in accidents.[17]

Some of the effects of hormones on memory and the brain can be attributed simply to the hot flashes and loss of sleep associated with menopause. Simply put, if you are losing sleep night after night, you are more likely to be forgetful, scatter-brained, and moody. Hormone replacement therapy, by helping to restore your normal sleep patterns, may also help restore your normal memory and moods.

However, studies suggest that estrogen has more direct effects on memory as well. Women who have had their ovaries and uterus surgically removed at a young age show "deficits in verbal memory," and restoring estrogen eliminates the deficit.[18]

In studies of nonmenopausal women, estrogen level changes during the menstrual cycle are associated with the enhancement of certain mental skills. For example, when estrogen levels are high, verbal fluency, the ability to articulate speech, and creativity all increase.[19]

These links between estrogen and mental or cognitive skills have encouraged doctors and scientists to study the potential of estrogen to prevent or treat Alzheimer's. As many as 10 clinical trials have evaluated the benefits of estrogen for women with Alzheimer's, and all have shown improvement in those women who took estrogen. Women who had only mild or moderate Alzheimer's fared better than those who already had severe dementia, and when treatment was stopped, the improvements went away.

There is also increasing evidence that estrogen therapy may significantly reduce the risk of *developing* Alzheimer's. Nine of ten recent studies have shown a significantly lower risk of Alzheimer's among estrogen users, anywhere from 35 percent to as much as 50 percent.[20]

The effects of estrogen—or lack of it—on the brain are not limited to Alzheimer's. Many women in early to midmenopause describe being in a "fog" which hangs over their brain, making them feel dull and unfocused. Women who have high-stress jobs or multiple responsibilities at home or work can suffer tremendously. Hormones are linked to moods and personality in ways we are usually not fully aware of. But those around you may notice changes in your personality or attitude that concern them and can affect your life in a negative way. These include depression, expressed either as sadness or "flat" emotions, irritability, confusion, or agitation.

Sleep disturbances can aggravate any of those symptoms. If you are not sleeping well because of hot flashes, your mood will definitely be diminished. Nor will it be helped by waking up at 3 A.M. or 4 A.M. every night and having trouble getting back to sleep, another very common effect of hormone deficiency. Sometimes the sleep problem is not waking, but getting poor quality sleep—when you wake up in the morning not feeling rested.

Hormone replacement therapy is terrific for symptoms like these, but needs to be carefully adjusted to limit the side effects. It does not necessarily take a large dose of hormone to correct these problems.

Depression

• • •

Another significant, and often hidden, cause of memory loss and some Alzheimer's-like effects is depression. By some estimates, as many as one woman in three have signs of depression. It is not uncommon in my practice to see women who are barely functional in their daily lives . . . yet they have put up with feeling bad because they simply cannot see a way out and believe they must bear it in silence. They assume that the stress in their lives (and who doesn't have stress?) is responsible and since they can't see how to eliminate their stress they're certainly not going to be able to eliminate their mood disturbances.

That's nonsense. There is no need to suffer when there are so many resources available, including hormonal therapy, antidepressants, motivational therapy, psychological support, and intervention. None are mutually exclusive.

Sometimes the stigma of having a problem prevents women from seeking help. Times have changed and so should we. As role models to our children, we must accept (and teach them to accept) treatment when it makes sense and can improve our quality of life. Nothing is more disturbing than the woman who is severely depressed, crying five times a day, and under no circumstances will consider an antidepressant... unless it's when I evaluate someone who is on tranquilizers, sleeping pills, and antidepressants without ever being checked for hormonal deficiencies by anyone.

Often, more than one approach may be needed, such as a combination of hormonal and antidepressant treatment. You must always have a hormonal assessment before an adequate treatment plan can be designed.

Note that what works well for one individual may not work at all for another. If you insist on taking another woman's pills, or imitating her regimen you're probably going to be dissatisfied. Women who do this frequently wind up abandoning treatment altogether—sometimes forever. That is why it is very important to work with a specialist in hormones, and to communicate with her about any negative side effects, so adjustments may be made in a timely fashion. It does require patience, particularly when dealing with brain dysfunction, because of the brain's sensitive nature and very individual response. When it comes to the brain, adjustments are often a matter of gradual process, not overnight improvement.

The good news is that the brain is resilient and can bounce back to premium function no matter how long you've experienced symptoms. In fact, it often responds so quickly that women have a hard time believing the improvement is related to their medication. However, if they experiment by discontinuing therapy, they soon realize the truth, because their original problems return just as rapidly as they'd disappeared!

Use It or Lose It

• • •

Aging and hormone deficiency do diminish our ability to learn, remember, process information, react, and move with coordination. The good news is that the brain ap-

> pears to respond to mental exercise. Challenging your brain on a daily basis, and continuing to stimulate your intellect, will help keep it sharp longer.

Now back to our doctor Sylvia. We started her on a low-dose estrogen patch called Vivelle, adding Prometrium (an oral progesterone) on a continuous regimen. When the adhesive on the patch caused some irritation, we simply had her rotate the places on her body where she applied it. Within four weeks, she was sleeping and concentrating noticeably better, and after six months, she reported a 70 percent improvement in memory and other brain functions. It also reassured her to know, since her mother has Alzheimer's, that her chances of contracting it herself will be reduced.

The Gospel Truth—THE BRAIN: "I'm Having More and More 'Senior Moments.' Could I Be Getting Alzheimer's."

• • •

1. Alzheimer's disease is a progressive disease of aging that affects one's ability to think, reason, and remember clearly. It may cause irritability, depression, and when severe, hallucinations and delusions. It can leave its victims entirely unable to care for themselves.
2. Nearly 50 percent of people over the age of 85 may be afflicted with some degree of brain dysfunction.
3. Estrogen has been shown to lower the risk of Alzheimer's disease and improve cognitive function.
4. Estrogen also may improve mental health by improving sleep, increasing memory capacity, and elevating mood.

12

INCONTINENCE
"I Lose Urine When I Cough or Sneeze, But I Am Embarrassed to Tell Anyone."

● ● ●

Corinne, a widowed 58-year-old executive assistant to the CEO of a pharmaceutical firm, told me:

"I was sitting at work one day, and I'd had a bad cold for a couple of weeks. And for the first time ever, when I was coughing rather hard, I lost a small amount of urine, which I could not control. Over the next six months, it became progressively worse, and now it's interfering with my lifestyle fairly significantly. It's particularly a problem when I work out at the gym during aerobics . . . even the slightest jarring motion and it will happen. I find myself emptying my bladder frequently to try and avoid it, and I'm afraid to drink too much liquid, in case it makes it worse. I've been reluctant to talk about it, because it's embarrassing, and there's probably not much I can do about it anyway. But I'm very concerned that it may get worse and prevent me from participating in even more activities. Is there anything that I can do?"

Uncontrolled urination and loss of urine are known as incontinence. Those who suffer from incontinence often suffer from embarrassment, discomfort, and even shame. Society tends to view anyone who is incontinent as feeble, senile, or otherwise mentally incompetent. Incontinent people will therefore often attempt to hide the problem, even from their doctors. They may avoid situations where they may laugh, or exercise in even the mildest form, or socializing in a group.

There are four main types of incontinence:

- Stress incontinence: leakage of urine caused by activity, such as sneezing, coughing, lifting something, or even climbing stairs.
- Urge incontinence: a sudden strong need to urinate, followed by uncontrollable loss.
- Mixture incontinence: a combination of stress and urge incontinence, sort of the worst of both worlds.
- Overflow incontinence: frequent or constant leakage of urine, similar to a leaky faucet, made worse when the bladder is full.

The number of Americans suffering from incontinence and related problems is estimated between 13 and 17 million. Women make up about 80 percent of these cases, and 20 to 25 percent are severe cases . . . the kind you can't ignore. The cost of managing this health-care problem, in terms of medical treatment and supplemental aids (such as adult diapers), etc., may be as much as $6 billion!

In younger women incontinence is most likely to be caused by multiple births, large babies, or chronic cough. Women are more prone to incontinence and related problems than men because their urethras are shorter, which makes them more accessible to bacteria and subsequent bladder infection. At any age incontinence can be triggered by diabetes, abdominal surgery (hysterectomy, etc.), nerve damage, certain medications, and pelvic organ prolapse. We're not helped by the body changes we typically experience as we age, including weight gain and the resulting changes in abdominal pressure.

In menopause, it may be caused by the drying of tissues and mucous membranes from low estrogen, which creates imbalances in the delicate pressure differential that controls the urinary flow. Menopause is also associated with impaired circulation and decreasing lubrication, which can be corrected by estrogen.

Additional symptoms and changes to the urogenital tract that may accompany incontinence and should be reported to your physician include the following:

1. Sandpaper-like irritation of the vaginal tissues and low moisture
2. Itching or burning of the vulva (external area)
3. Pain or discomfort during sexual activity (dyspareunia)
4. The need to urinate more frequently with small amounts of urine (called frequency) or the need to urinate more urgently (called—guess what?—urgency)

There may be aggravating factors that increase or mimic symptoms of incontinence, such as:

• bladder infection
• yeast infections
• bacterial vaginosis
• trichomoniasis (a parasitic infection)
• sexually transmitted diseases, including chlamydia
• allergies
• douching
• certain inflammatory bowel diseases
• irritation from tampons or birth-control devices
• skin conditions, such as eczema or psoriasis

During menopause, the vagina becomes shortened and less able to stretch without injury. The texture of the vagina changes as well, with fewer natural folds. The lubricating fluid produced by the tissue decreases, contributing to discomfort during sex and while urinating. Itching, burning, and an increased tendency toward breaks in the skin and bleeding are often the result.

Because of both the location and the shortness of the urethra, women are more prone than men to bacterial contamination and infection. Sexual activity can aggravate this, as can certain habits, such as "holding" urine. Lack of estrogen may cause the urethra's tissue to dry out, additionally increasing the likelihood and severity of these infections, and contributing further to the discomfort associated with incontinence. Any suspicion of a urinary-tract infection should be investigated by analysis and culture and treated early.

Hormone replacement therapy can slow down and reverse some incontinence because there are many estrogen receptors in the female urethra and urinary tract tissue. Estrogen increases "urethral vascular perfusion," or the health of and blood flow to the vessels in the area. Restoring the suppleness of the vaginal tissue improves urogenital tract health. Estrogen also seems to benefit the muscles involved. Note that oral estrogen does not relieve incontinence; it has to be applied locally to the vaginal area.

Estring, a vaginal ring, is one such treatment. The ring is placed in the vagina like a diaphragm, and releases small amounts of estrogen over a three-month period. (It does not interfere with sex.) Estring is great for women who want a very low dose of estrogen, delivered continuously without the messiness of creams and lotions. Other women may prefer local creams that are used two or three times a week. This is a better choice for those who are taking oral or patch hormone replacement therapy for other menopausal symptoms.

Stress incontinence can be treated by phenyl-propanolamine or pseudoephedrine, while urge incontinence can be helped with oxybutrimin or propantheline. The drugs imipramine, doceprin, desipramine, and nortryptyline have also been used with some success. A urology evaluation will determine the best course of action.

Finally, there are new devices being developed and tested that plug the urethra and support the bladder neck. One is a small foam tab that temporarily covers the urethra. It is not as unpleasant as it sounds, and seems to be much less uncomfortable than adult diapers.

In addition to any of these therapies, Kegel exercises will help maximize your benefits. In some cases, they may be *all* that is needed. The Kegel exercise is a simple tensing, or contracting, of the muscle that controls bladder flow. Lightly tense the muscle as if you are trying to stop the flow of urine, hold it for a few seconds, then release. Do this about ten times, several times during the course of a day. (In bodybuilder's lingo, you may want to do six sets of ten reps a day.) You'll notice improvement within a month.

Kegel exercises can be practiced anywhere: in the car, sitting at your desk, standing in line at the market. (If you're grimacing and making faces, you're tensing too hard. And unlike at the gym, grunting and counting off the reps is probably not socially acceptable.) These exercises may also have the pleasant side effect of improving sexual response and possibly even orgasmic intensity. They may also be used to increase your partner's pleasure. (Kegel exercises may be practiced by men as well, resulting in similar benefits.)

Our evaluation of Corinne began with a physical examination, which revealed dry, atrophied vaginal tissues, and a urine culture, which was positive for bacteria. We treated her infection with antibiotics, instructed her on Kegel exercises, and started her on ¼ applicator of estrogen cream inserted into the vagina three to four times a week. She was urged to void frequently, especially prior to vigorous activity. We also recommended a water-soluble lubricant be used during intercourse. Twelve months later, she is doing well with very few episodes of urine loss. She is surprised and relieved to have her life back.

The Gospel Truth—INCONTINENCE: "I Lose Urine When I Cough or Sneeze, but I am Embarrassed to Tell Anyone."

• • •

1. The uncontrolled loss of urine is known as incontinence.
2. Stress incontinence is a loss of urine caused by activity or pressure within the abdomen. It is especially likely to occur during coughing, sneezing, laughing, and vigorous exercise.
3. It is estimated as many as 17 million Americans suffer from incontinence and related problems.
4. One of the causes of incontinence is the drying of tissues and mucous membranes, which creates imbalances in the pressure differential that controls the urinary flow.

5. Women are more prone to incontinence and related problems than men because their urethra is shorter, which makes it more accessible to bacteria and subsequent bladder infection.

6. Hormone therapy can slow down the worsening of incontinence and can greatly improve mild cases.

13

MENOPAUSE AND SEXUALITY
The Difference Between Getting Hot and Being Hot

• • •

Carol, a 48-year-old marketing executive, came to my office for a wellness physical. Upon reviewing her questionnaire, I noticed she had written, "severe decrease in sex drive." When I asked her about this, she said:

"I really love my fiancé, and I feel close to him in almost every way possible. He's a caring man, and I know he isn't the problem. But for some reason, I still just have absolutely no interest in sex. I don't understand it! When we started dating three years ago, my sex drive was really healthy. I've always been very positive about sex, initiated it, and really enjoyed it, but about a year ago it was just as though someone turned the faucet off, and it was gone. I find it really disturbing, and I'm sure Bill thinks I'm just not interested in him anymore. It's hurting his feelings, and he can't believe it's not him."

When I asked if Carol had noticed any other symptoms of menopause, such as hot flashes, she said no, but she mentioned she had felt a moderate amount of vaginal dryness, which also made her more reluctant to participate in sexual activity. "Do you think I'm just losing interest in sex because I'm getting old?" she asked.

Come on: women of this age are not old! But the fact is, changes in sex drive rank among the top five reasons women seek a physician's counsel for menopause (along with fatigue, hot flashes, sleep trouble, and, what was the fifth one again? Oh yeah, memory loss).

There are significant chemical changes in the brain that affect sex drive at this stage of life, as well as physical changes, like less vaginal elasticity. Primarily, though, the major cause of changes in sex drive at this stage of life are changes in estrogen and androgen levels, and they may be treated with testosterone.

Before treating the physical symptoms, though, it is important for a physician and patient to understand the psychological and emotional components of libido. While *sex* is physical, *sexuality* is a complex blend of the emotional, physical, and chemical.

Cultural Predisposition and Attitudes

Sexual drive generally decreases gradually in both men and women as they age. This does not mean an abrupt halt, and the rate of any extent of decreased interest is individual and of varying importance.

So much of our attitude about sex in our middle-aged years and beyond has to do with the way our culture perceives such behavior. While middle-aged men have been (and perhaps still are) encouraged to continue to be sexually active to demonstrate their virility and potency, middle-aged women are tacitly encouraged to accept less sexual activity. Women who find themselves single owing to death of a spouse or divorce may have stopped seeing themselves as sexual beings just because they don't have a partner. They may be afraid to become sexually active from fear of AIDS and other transmissible diseases, which probably didn't pose a risk the last time they were out dating.

Other factors that may affect a woman's interest in sex (or lack thereof) are:

- illness of herself or her partner
- loss of a partner through death or divorce
- for women without partners, a decreased availability of new partners
- loss of privacy or sexual freedom, either because of adult children or elderly parents living at home, or residence in a re-

tirement home (something you may not think about at the time you move into one)

For some women of this age, moral issues of sex and marriage also come into play. A woman may feel it is wrong to have sex outside of marriage, yet may be hesitant to marry for fear of losing social security benefits and other income. She may be reluctant to enter any relationship due to bad past experiences.

Certain drugs decrease libido and sexual response, including the delay or complete loss of orgasm. Examples include:

- Blood pressure medicines, such as MAO inhibitors
- Narcotics such as heroin and methadone
- Alcohol
- Antidepressants such as Prozac, Zoloft, and others
- Tagamet

Previous attitudes often correlate with a woman's view of her sexuality as she ages. In general women who enjoyed sex in their younger years will continue to do so during and beyond midlife, while those who have not enjoyed sex previously may view any reduction in sexual activity as a relief rather than a loss. Partners may also lose interest in sex or have decreased capacity for sexual activity. Indeed, some women and their partners may simply have never learned satisfactory "technical skills": A surprisingly large number of people have never realized full function and satisfaction in a sexual relationship! It is never too late to start learning, and you may be much better at it this time.

On the other hand, not all women lose interest in sex; some menopausal women have an increased interest in sex, possibly because there's no more fear of getting pregnant. In addition, their sexual response may be more intense and pleasurable.

Testosterone

Testosterone, as we've discussed, is a "male" hormone, or androgen, that contributes to libido, or sexual desire. Like estrogen, androgen levels decrease during menopause. Increasing your testosterone in the presence of inadequate estrogen levels may be ineffective. It is the balance of all the hormones, rather than the level of any one, that makes for vibrant health. When women visit our center complaining of low sex drive, even though they are on testosterone, we often find their estrogen levels to be very low.

Testosterone comes in many forms:

- Mixed compounds, such as Estratest, in which estrogen and testosterone are blended together.
- Testosterone lozenges.
- Testosterone creams. These are recommended for women who prefer not to or can't take oral medication.
- Injections. Physicians and patients try to avoid these, because administration is inconvenient, but they may be useful if a woman can't use other reasonable options. Woman can and do inject themselves if necessary.

See Appendix A for more information on dosages and forms.

Besides the increase in libido (sex drive), benefits of testosterone include decreased breast tenderness and an increase in energy, feelings of well-being, and sexuality. (We distinguish here between sex drive—desiring sex—and sexuality, which includes sex drive, sexual performance, attitude—the "entire works.")

Also, like estrogen, testosterone is thought to stimulate bone formation, and slow bone resorption, thereby helping to prevent osteoporosis.

Testosterone may also improve age-related memory and attention deficits. Researchers are studying the positive effects of androgens on Alzheimer's-related cognitive impairments, and also its relationship with immunology and insulin physiology in the aging.

Negative side effects of testosterone, though less likely when you use low doses, include "virilization": hair growth, voice changes, acne, irritability, and hostile behavior.

There's been some discussion in the press and medical community of unfavorable effects of androgens on lipids or HDL/LDL (high-density lipoprotein/low-density lipoprotein) balance, where favorable cholesterol seems to become unfavorable. However, the effect is not significant at the very low doses used in this type of therapy.

Finally, it must be said that testosterone is not the only factor affecting sexuality during the menopause years. In the next few pages, we will discuss areas that all deserve attention when treating sex-related complaints. Other symptoms of menopause, as well as their treatments, may affect sexuality directly or indirectly.

Urinary Tract and Bladder Issues

Menopausal and perimenopausal women often lose sexual desire because of vaginal dryness and tearing of the vulvar/vaginal tissue, loss of lubrication, and/or burning. Allergy pills and other types of antihistamine may cause drying of the vaginal tissue, making your problem worse. Birth-control pills can do this as well. By no means should you or your partner assume that your dryness is a result of not being "turned on" (sexually aroused).

Sexual intercourse may cause damage to the urethra and irritate dry tissue, both of which increase the likelihood of bacterial infections. You may have incontinence as an unwanted bonus. On top of the embarrassment, which isn't going to do anything for your sex drive, incontinence can cause the skin to become further irritated, sore, and cracked. In some cases, a woman's skin and internal tissues may take on a rough, "sandpaper" texture, which can make the rubbing of your undergarments when you walk, or even prolonged sitting, very uncomfortable. Although low levels of estrogen are usually the problem, biopsies of this area are needed to rule out more serious causes, especially when there is abnormal bleeding and/or a higher risk factor for uterine cancer.

Painful Sex

Another common consequence of low estrogen is painful sex, or dyspareunia. It is estimated that 25 percent of women over the age of 40 suffer from this malady. The figure increases to 50 percent of women over 50 and 60 percent of women over 60. Dyspareunia may result from tears in the tissue and accompanying bleeding, from skin irritation and rashes (dermatitis), especially on the vulva and buttocks, and from failure to use lubrication or adequately lubricate naturally during sex. Endometriosis or other problems affecting the internal organs can also be the culprit.

Incontinence can be treated, as discussed earlier, through local estrogen application and Kegel exercises. Estrogen cream applied topically also works to restore suppleness, flexibility, and moisture to vaginal tissues. Improvement of vaginal dryness occurs steadily for up to 24 months after starting either oral or local estrogen therapy. It can restore proper function to 90 percent of the women who take it, and may return vaginal resilience to the level a woman enjoyed prior to turning 40. And don't worry: the small doses of estrogen in the cream will not affect a male partner. In any case, you can use it 45 minutes prior to sex, so it will be fully absorbed.

Minor vaginal dryness can also be treated with estrogen, for example by the use of lubricants such as Astroglide, K-Y jelly, Lubrin, and many newer products, alone or in addition to cream. "Vaginal moisturizers," such as Replens and K-Y Long Lasting, do more than coat the surface to make it slippery; they actually work to make the tissue less dry. Foaming lubricants, such as Transilube, mimic natural secretions fairly well. Vitamin E oil, which comes in little capsules, can be used for lubrication, and helps some women relieve itching, local burning, and irritation.

Any product you use (with the exception of vitamin E) should be water-soluble (dissolve easily in water), and should be especially designed for this purpose. No WD-40 allowed! Ingredients such as alcohol, perfumes, or petroleum jelly (as in Vaseline®) cause local irritation, and increase the risk of infection in the vagina and bladder. Alcohol and petroleum-based products may also damage condoms and diaphragms, which decreases their protection. Avoid placing large amounts of lubricant near the urethra, where urine drains from the bladder. (A small amount, which is unavoidable, won't hurt.) Bacteria introduced into the lubricant containers with use can contaminate these compounds. Check the containers frequently for discoloration or odor, and discard if there's any doubt.

Lubricants are temporary solutions to the problem of vaginal dryness. They work by covering the symptom without treating the underlying cause. Still, they are a relief from discomfort, and can be used while waiting for more effective therapies to take effect, or if other options are unavailable.

Sleep

Sleep disturbances, such as those brought on by hot flashes, night sweats, or depression will make women tired and irritable. As previously discussed, hot flashes and depression may be reduced with hormone or other therapy, which in turn may reduce the sleep disturbances. But left untreated, what happens to sexual desire when you're tired and irritable? You've got it—it drops.

In addition, insomnia increases during the menopause. Sleep fragmentation, which occurs when your sleep is frequently interrupted during the night, is common. Women who have hot flashes may wake up as frequently as every eight minutes, but even those who don't have flashes can wake every 18 minutes. These are short awakenings that you rarely remember but leave you tired the next morning.

Another cause of sleep fragmentation is central sleep apnea, a condition in which you stop breathing periodically for 10 seconds or more, prompting you to wake up. These incidents may occur as many as 25 times a night. Various medications may help, such as Clonidine. Hormone replacement therapy seems to help as well.

Surgery

Surgery can reduce libido, for both physiological and psychological reasons. Physical reasons include fatigue from the surgical procedure, and (in the case of surgery on the reproductive organs) possible resulting hormone imbalance. In general, surgically induced menopause may lessen sexual desire more severely.

From a psychological perspective, a woman's perception of her body is an important component of her sexual health. Self-esteem can be difficult to maintain as we age under the best of circumstances—and more so in the face of breast surgery or other visual changes due to surgery or illness—making a woman feel less sexual and less interested in sex.

Following the removal of a breast or uterus, women may feel unattractive, and may avoid initiating sexual encounters. Their partners may treat them as less sexual, either from fear that sexual intercourse will cause pain or discomfort, or of looking at scars or other body changes. When either partner has a serious illness or is recuperating from one, pain, fear, or simple preoccupation may decrease desire. The fear of dying may overwhelm all other responses, even if not discussed.

It is important to have psychiatric counseling and support prior to major surgeries or treatments. This will allow you, your therapist, and physician to make a plan that will carry you through recovery. Whenever possible, it is recommended you see a counselor with your partner.

Hysterectomy deserves special mention here: Losing the uterus should not mean losing desire. Physical sensations may change, becoming better or just . . . different. Some women enjoy sex more, because they've gotten relief from menstrual or premenstrual pain or bleeding, or because they don't have to worry about getting pregnant.[21] On the other hand, if surgery is done inappropriately, without proper counseling, it may have a devastating impact. In general, if ovaries are removed or injured and the subsequent hormone decline is treated, significant problems will be prevented.

Interactions with Other Medication

Many medications—such as those for high blood pressure and depression—can also interfere with sexual desire. For example, the antidepressants Prozac and Zoloft can flatten or decrease sex drive. However, these medications are sometimes being taken for menopausal symptoms that might be better treated by hormone replacement. In that case, the solution may be simple: switch to hormones. When antidepressants *are* necessary, trying other formulas may lessen the problems.

Other Areas to Explore

Being with the wrong partner can decrease or eliminate sexual drive. If you are mistreated, physically or emotionally, or simply no longer connect on a "chemical" or intellectual level, no amount of hormones will fix it. If you suffer from shadows of former sexual abuse of any kind, get help to resolve those issues and move on with your life. You deserve to be happy, and to have a normal sex life.

Vibrators can be helpful in perimenopause and menopause for women who have delayed or incomplete orgasms. Experiment with the types and frequency of vibration to discover what enhances your sexual responses. Practice makes perfect, so go slow and work at it.

As mentioned in the chapter on incontinence, Kegel exercises may not only improve tissue tone and bladder control, but may also improve sexual response and orgasm. Practicing Kegel exercises daily is simple, can be done almost anywhere, and shows results in a relatively short time.

Don't Touch That! You Don't Know Where It's Been! (Menopause and Sexually Transmitted Diseases)

The menopause creates numerous challenges, not the least of which may be entering the singles life after divorce or the death of a spouse. With all the new risks of sexually transmitted disease, at least one of which is deadly, it can be awkward and frightening. We will attempt to cover the basics of the more common problems and dispel some myths.

"Sexually transmitted disease" (STD) or "venereal disease" (VD) as it was once commonly known (there are many slang terms you may know as well) creates a serious stigma for many people. Many of these conditions are very common and if you are sexually active with anyone other than yourself, you will be at some risk. Condoms and other barriers help protect you, but are by no means 100 percent effective.

Some viruses live in healthy tissue, and have long waiting times in a "carrier" state. People who are carriers may transmit harmful bacteria, viruses, and other pathogens without knowing they are sources of infection. There are also unethical individuals who knowingly put a partner at risk.

Some of the more common problems that sexually active people are at risk for include the following:

- Yeast Infections
  Yeast infections are benign fungal infections usually treated with creams or pills. They are commonly noticed as an itchy discharge, usually thick and clumpy. They can also start as a red, bumpy, itchy rash around the genitals, on the thighs, or even under the breasts. Yeast infections may be diagnosed by analysis of a vaginal discharge if present under the microscope. Yeast infections are not sexually transmitted diseases, per se, but they may occasionally cause fine, red bumps on a male partner's skin from contact. Men do not typically contract yeast infections; occasionally they are carriers. The over-the-counter creams work and are safe for treating the rash or the discharge. Desitin ointment or cornstarch is helpful to keep irritated areas dry while they heal, and to prevent further problems.
- Herpes
  Herpes is a sexually transmitted virus that lives in healthy nerve tissue. Infection is very, very painful on the first breakout, and forms one or more ulcerlike lesions. The breakout will recur, either frequently or infrequently, and usually flares up in the same area, such as the vulva, thigh, or buttocks. This virus is in the same family as the virus that causes cold sores. There are antiviral treatment and suppression regimens that prevent shedding of the virus and breakouts. Although herpes is treatable, it is not curable. Stress can increase breakouts, as can the time just before your period. Herpes is most infective when the lesions are present. At least a million new cases are reported each year.
- Chlamydia
  Chlamydia is an STD whose symptoms are so subtle, many women do not realize they have it. Its only symptom may be a slight vaginal discharge. Men are more likely to exhibit symptoms, such as penile discharge and pain while urinating. If left untreated, chlamydia can cause fallopian-tube damage resulting in infertility. It is diagnosed with a culture (a small

sample of discharge is taken and observed in the laboratory) and treated with antibiotics. There are approximately 3 million cases reported each year. If you haven't been tested and are at risk, you can ask to be tested on your next doctor's visit.

- Gonorrhea

  There are approximately 650,000 reported new cases of gonorrhea each year. Both partners need to be treated at the same time with antibiotics if either partner is diagnosed. Gonorrhea increases your risk of fallopian-tube damage, which can cause problems getting pregnant as well as a higher risk of having a tubal pregnancy. It also appears to increase the risk of contracting HIV. It is diagnosed by a simple vaginal culture. Symptoms of gonorrhea range from none to prominent discharges.

- Syphilis

  Syphilis and gonorrhea have both declined sharply in recent years, but still remain more prevalent in the United States than anywhere else in the developed world. Syphilis is diagnosed by a blood test called VDRL, and again, both partners have to be treated with antibiotics if either is infected. If left untreated, syphilis can lead to serious neurological problems and death. The main symptom is usually a large ulcer on the genitals.

- HIV/AIDS

  HIV (human immunodeficiency virus) is the virus that causes AIDS (acquired immune deficiency syndrome). It is detected by a blood test. The disease is deadly and can be spread by people who show no symptoms. The majority of women now living with AIDS contracted it from heterosexual contact, often from sharing needles with intravenous drug users. One of the most common early signs of HIV in women is frequent yeast infections. (Of course, getting frequent yeast infections doesn't necessarily mean you are HIV-positive! There are many other possible reasons.) As the disease progresses, your immune system loses its ability to fight disease, and you become likely to develop secondary, "opportunistic" infections like pneumonia, and certain rare cancers, like Kaposi's sarcoma. By 1996, HIV/AIDS was the fourth leading cause of death among women aged 25–44. There is no cure but a variety of therapies are helping people live longer and better lives. The only protection against this disease is abstinence, followed in effectiveness by the male condom. Any method of protection is more effective in combination with spermicide.

- Condyloma (venereal warts)

  There are as many as 80 versions of this virus, which often appear as itchy or painful external warts or patches of skin. It also can appear as viral injury of the genital tissues in the form of an abnormal Pap smear or abnormal vulvar skin biopsy. A large percentage of the population (perhaps 15 percent) carries the virus. There are 5.5 million cases reported each year and many more that probably aren't tracked. It can be spread by an unknowing partner who does not demonstrate any signs or symptoms, and it may even lie dormant for years. This results in varying intervals before the time of acquiring the virus and demonstrating any sign of it. In fact, you may never exhibit any symptoms. Some types may result in increased risk of certain genital cancers, including cancer of the cervix. It is diagnosed by visual inspection and/or biopsy. Condyloma is treated by medication, or removal by various techniques. There is no cure but it is usually a manageable condition.

- Bacterial Vaginosis

  Bacterial vaginosis is an infection that causes a gray discharge and the infamous "fishy" odor. It is diagnosed by viewing a sample of the discharge under a microscope, and by measuring the pH (acidity/alkalinity) of the vagina. It may be treated with metronidazole or ampicillin. In certain conditions a male partner can become infected and require treatment.

- Trichomoniasis

  Trichomoniasis is a parasitic infection. As many as 5 million cases are reported annually. Trichomoniasis is also diagnosed by examining a sample of discharge under a microscope. It is treated with metronidazole. Trichomoniasis can increase the risk of contracting HIV. It also is known for little red dots on the cervix and vagina when viewed at examination.

Barrier-type contraceptives—primarily male and female condoms—can help protect against most sexually transmitted diseases, if used properly. The addition of spermicides increases the degree of protection. Birth-control pills do not offer any protection from STDs at all.

It should be noted that most of these diseases can be transmitted to unborn children during delivery if left untreated. With good supervision, this complication can be avoided.

Hepatitis B (and other types of hepatitis) may also be spread through sexual contact. It may not be curable in some cases; however, there is a vaccine against it. Some people may be carriers of the disease. I recommend the vaccination for everybody, particularly health-care professionals and others who may come into contact with blood.

Women experience "bumps" all through their lives in various places on their bodies. Mysterious bumps on the vulva or in the vagina bring anxious thoughts of at least three undesirables: herpes, venereal warts, or cancer. Fortunately, you will be wrong a lot of the time. Bumps and other symptoms may be caused by inflammation, skin rashes, allergies, blocked hair follicles, benign cysts, and genetic predisposition. Often we take a first look at ourselves with a mirror to investigate a bump, and think *something* looks very wrong or resembles a bad thing we've heard about. If we don't have anything to compare it with (maybe you've never looked before), it can be quite scary. Some of our internal and external sexual organs are normally quite irregular in look and feel, but completely normal. No two are alike, either, so your friends can't help you.

If something seems wrong to you, it should be evaluated by a professional, especially if it is burning, itching, painful, or different in some distinct way. Even if it is nothing, your resulting peace of mind is worth it. In general, an old bump that's the same for years does not have as much importance as

- a new, growing bump
- one that changes color
- one that bleeds
- one that doesn't heal

Discharges can be white, yellow, green, blood-tinged, gray, or clear, to name a few. Not all discharge from the vagina is abnormal, and the "quality" of a woman's secretions may vary during the month—from very little to watery, clear and "stretchy," to thick white—and still be normal.

Pregnancy

Many menopausal and perimenopausal women can't wait to stop using birth control. They feel a great sense of freedom at being able to have sex without worry of pregnancy, and this may actually lead to an increase in their sex drive and sexual enjoyment. But be careful: you can't assume that when menopause symptoms start you are infertile. An egg can slip through, and we encounter a postbiblical Sarah who has a child in her late 40s or even later, despite many clear symptoms of being in menopause. (As it says in the Bible, "It had ceased to be with Sarah, after the manner of women.")

Lack of egg production can be determined by measuring follicle stimulating hormone over a period of time, and/or no period for six months. Until your doctor verifies lack of egg production, it is a good idea to continue using birth control. Many women will find the choices available much wider than when they were younger. Available birth control methods include:

- Sterilization, such as tubal ligation for women or vasectomy for men; otherwise known as "having your tubes tied." Tubal ligation is an in-hospital procedure and has all the risks of any surgery. Vasectomy is done in an office setting and is less risky.
- Barrier methods include the diaphragm, condom—male and female, cervical cap, and spermicides.
- Hormonal methods, such as birth-control pills, Depo-Provera (long-term injection) and Norplant (under-the-skin implant).
- Intrauterine devices, or IUDs. These small devices inserted into the uterus by your doctor prevent an egg from implanting in the uterine wall by making the environment less favorable. There is an increased risk of infection with these.

- "Russian roulette," such as rhythm or withdrawal. Rhythm is logical, but difficult to do with accuracy, especially when your period is no longer occurring at regular intervals. This is one birth-control plan with no room for error!

Of the above methods, only the male condom has been reliable (although not 100 percent effective) against sexually transmitted disease, including AIDS/HIV. Even if you are using one of the other methods of birth control, use of a condom is recommended to protect against these venereal diseases.

Back to our patient Carol, and her severely decreased sex drive: We put Carol on Estratest (a brand of estrogen-testosterone combination therapy) and a local estrogen cream. Since she had previously had a hysterectomy, we didn't have to put her on progesterone. We monitored her for side effects, which we familiarized her with prior to starting. In about four weeks, her sexual drive and function began to return, but she had increased acne and some irritability. We alternated her Estratest with plain estrogen every other day to lower the testosterone dosage as maintenance. She will be checked every two months for six to 12 months for dosage adjustments, by reviewing her journals and blood testing as indicated. Alternate sources of testosterone can be tried as well to minimize side effects.

The Gospel Truth—MENOPAUSE AND SEXUALITY: The Difference Between Getting Hot and Being Hot

• • •

1. Just because a woman is beginning menopause does not mean she is old, nor does it mean she must or should give up sex.
2. Sex drive is affected during menopause by changes in brain chemistry, lower hormone levels, and physiological changes, such as vaginal dryness.
3. The "male" hormone testosterone may help restore libido, or sexual desire, in women who have lost their

sex drive during the menopause. It requires estrogen levels to work and is not for everybody.

4. The blend of estrogen, progesterone, and testosterone together must be balanced for the optimum results.

5. Positive side effects of testosterone may include reduced hot flashes, an increase in energy, increased feeling of well-being, decreased breast tenderness, as well as increased sex drive and sexual performance.

6. More research is needed, but there is some evidence that testosterone may have positive effects on osteoporosis, Alzheimer's, immunology, and insulin physiology.

7. Negative side effects of testosterone include "virilization," which causes hair growth, voice changes, acne, and/or irritability and hostile behavior. These are uncommon with low-dose therapy. There has been some evidence that higher doses may have unfavorable effects on cholesterol balance.

8. Other menopause-related issues that may affect sexuality include urinary-tract problems, progesterone deficiency, sleep deficiency, surgery, and interactions with other medication.

9. Being with the wrong partner may defeat any and all treatments. Heal thyself.

10. Sexually transmitted diseases know no age limits—practice safe sex regardless of your hormone levels.

11. Pregnancy may still be a concern during perimenopause. Take proper precautions until you are sure your body has stopped producing eggs.

14

SIDE EFFECTS
The Good, the Bad and the Ugly

● ● ●

Shawna, a 56-year-old single woman with no high cancer risk factors in her personal health history and six failed estrogen trials, told me:

"I don't care what you suggest, I've probably already had it. They all make my breasts feel like painful watermelons. I can't sleep on my stomach and can't stand being touched. I'm here for one last try because I've read a lot about the benefits and don't want to be left out! Frankly, though, I doubt you can help me."

Unfortunately, there can be side effects to hormone replacement therapy, including breast tenderness, bleeding, stomach upset, skin-pigmentation changes, weight gain, fluid retention, allergies, and headache. In most cases, these side effects are not serious, medically speaking. Nevertheless, they are "serious" in that they stop people from taking hormone replacement therapy, and expose them to greater risk of heart disease, osteoporosis, Alzheimer's, and colon cancer.

Negative side effects of the three significant hormones include the following:

Estrogen
- Bloating
- Irregular bleeding

- Breast tenderness
- Blood clots
- Gallbladder problems
- Fibroid enlargement
- Skin pigmentation
- Anxiety

Progesterone

- Moodiness and irritability
- Depression
- Bloating
- Abnormal bleeding
- Increased oily skin
- Acne or other skin disruptions
- Frizzy hair
- Headaches
- Breast pain
- PMS

Testosterone

- Increased facial and body hair
- Deepening of voice
- Increased aggression
- Too much sex drive
- Oily skin
- Acne
- Irritability

Additionally, any of the three hormones may result in stomach upset, allergy, rash, swelling, weight gain, and hair changes.

Positive effects of the three significant hormones include the following:

Estrogen

- Improved quality of sleep
- Improved mood
- Better quality skin, hair, and nails
- Improved libido
- Improved vaginal lubrication
- Decrease in musculoskeletal aches and pains
- Elimination of hot flashes and night sweats
- Improvement of mental functioning

Progesterone

- Suppression of endometriosis
- Potential increase of sex drive
- Control of abnormal bleeding
- Improvement in mood
- Bone protection
- Reduced hot flashes

Testosterone

- Improved sense of well-being
- Improved elasticity and resilience of vaginal tissues
- Improved libido
- Improved sexual performance
- Control of difficult-to-suppress hot flashes

Many of these hormones can work in two different directions, depending on individual response and on the dosage. For example, properly dosed progesterone can control abnormal bleeding, while improperly dosed progesterone can make it worse.

Most patients who tell me they have tried "everything" usually haven't, although I understand how it may feel like it when several options in a row fail for you, or when a professional mistakenly tells you there *are* no more options. I suggest patients prepare a detailed list of dates, dosages, types of hormone replacement, side effects, and amount of time to develop them. All of these details are critical. More than a few patients were told (or told me) they were on the "lowest dose" of a hormone when they were not.

Some "side effects," such as bleeding, are actually signs of serious underlying conditions. Abnormal uterine bleeding in a woman over 40 may be a sign of fibroids, polyps, infection, hormone imbalance, adenomyosis (a benign disease of the uterus), or premalignant disease. Less commonly, it can be a sign of genital-tract cancer—of the vulva, vagina, cervix, uterus, or, even less commonly, ovary. It must be evaluated properly before any conclusions can be drawn.

A simple office endometrial sample, or biopsy, with the newer small flexible catheters will clarify if any problem exists: The pathologist looks at a small piece of tissue under the microscope and tells us what treatment direction to go in. Ultrasound is also helpful in identifying a cause and especially to evaluate the thickness of the uterine lining, which is what is shed when we bleed. It can also be used to screen for problems in a woman who displays no symptoms but is at high risk of uterine lining diseases, including cancer. An example would be a woman on tamoxifen.

SIDE EFFECTS

Bloating: Water retention or bloating is another complaint that can be treated in several different ways. Lowering salt intake is important because salt helps the body to retain water. If lowering your dietary salt intake doesn't work, or you are already on a low-salt diet, a mild diuretic is the next step. This can be as mild as a cup of tea, and can be stepped up to include prescription diuretics if the problem warrants it. Although coffee and other strong caffeine drinks are diuretics, they can have other side effects (like jitters) and should not be taken to excess. Lowering or changing the progestin dose may also help, as progestin sometimes seems to affect bloating more so than estrogen.

Weight gain: Nobody wants or needs it. Unfortunately, hormones are blamed for a great many weight problems they don't deserve. Frequently, a woman's lifestyle and metabolism contribute to a slow increase in weight, regardless of hormone usage. This is borne out by the fact that many women quit their hormone therapy yet the weight gain rarely goes away. Often, unsupportive partners make the problem worse. What role *do* hormones play? Too much hormone may cause weight gain, water retention, or tenderness, but when properly adjusted, this is usually not a problem. The type of hormone and dosage can have an effect that can be managed with careful attention. Don't let the possibility of weight gain alone make you lose out on the many benefits of hormone therapy, because the potential weight gain can often be minimized or avoided entirely through adjustments in your replacement regimen.

Often when treating women who have gained weight, I discover that not all of the gain is due to menopause or hormone therapy. Entering hormone therapy is often a good time to review and modify your diet. Keeping a food diary may be helpful to track your calorie intake, which your doctor can then help determine if appropriate for your age and size. As you age, your metabolism changes, and a diet that was fine for you in the past may no longer be appropriate. Speaking of metabolism, exercise designed to burn calories and fat as well as increase the metabolic rate is invaluable and increases your overall health. Join a weight-loss program if you have trouble maintaining a diet or exercise program alone.

Breast tenderness: This is a common complaint when there is too *little,* as well as too *much,* estrogen or progesterone. (Fibrocystic breast change can make the tenderness even worse.) Taking 800 to 1,000 IU (international units) of vitamin E can be very helpful, along with the restriction of caffeine. These interventions are controversial because scientific proof is difficult to obtain, but in practice they seem to be helpful. Progesterone compounds cause breast tenderness more often than estrogen does, and adjusting the dosage or type of compound may help.

Adjusting your dosage will be very successful in most cases. Particularly if you are over 60 when you start hormones, your breast tissue may be too painful on normal doses. Your breasts just can't handle the changes after a long absence of estrogen. Additional relief may be found by decreasing the salt in your diet.

GI problems: Gastrointestinal problems such as nausea or stomach pain may be a result of the binding agents or dye in hormone pills, of a too-high dose, or of the hormones themselves. Changing brands or trying an alternate route such as the patch or cream can combat this very effectively. An allergic reaction to the medication itself may be dealt with this way, depending on severity. Hormones derived from animal sources may cause allergies that are not a problem with plant sources and vice versa.

Headache: Migraine headaches in particular can result from changes in the levels of estrogen or progesterone (most often progesterone). If they began in the perimenopausal years, a deficiency of estrogen is likely the culprit. If they begin after initiating treatment, they may be hormonally induced or aggravated, this can be from too much or too little of any of the hormones utilized in replacement, or an imbalance between any two components of treatment. Headaches associated with PMS-type symptoms are probably due to progesterone. Switching from cyclic to continuous regimen therapy is usually the best course of action, although for some women already on continuous therapy, switching to cyclic therapy may reduce the headaches. Generally speaking, the less change and the more level the hormones, the less they trigger headache.

As with breast tenderness and bloating, lowering your salt intake may also help headaches. Change the type or dose of estrogen or progestin; for example, consider a nonoral estrogen regimen such as a patch. The mechanisms that cause headaches are not entirely understood, so sometimes a small adjustment works wonders.

An interesting side note is that women who used to experience regular headaches around the time of their periods will often stop having headaches after starting hormone replacement therapy or from just the menopause itself. There are also many wonderful new treatment regimens for migraine and its variants that can be utilized in conjunction with hormonal balance therapy.

Depression: It is important for women undergoing HRT to have a good relationship with their doctors. Depression can "sneak up" on you, and you may not even realize it is related to your therapy, especially if there are many other changes occurring in your life. If you are taking progestin cyclically, try switching to continuous. If you are taking continuous, switch to cyclic. Every woman's body handles it differently, and the full effect is not predictable. Sometimes, it is advisable to take a "hormone holiday," and see if it is in fact the cause. If you stop taking the hormones and the depression persists, other causes should be examined. Measure your hormone levels to see if they are adequate. If you're on birth-control pills, try another with decreased progesterone/androgen levels.

Nausea: If taking pills makes you want to throw up, you are not alone. Some people have problems with even the mildest pills, either because they have sensitive stomachs, or because they are allergic to the active or inactive substances in the pill. There are a number of ways to attack this side effect. First, try taking the tablets at bedtime, and/or with meals. Mornings are sometimes a more stressful time of the day for us, and the stomach may be more sensitive. Next, try a non-oral product, such as a patch or gel, which may eliminate the problem entirely. Especially if you had a sensitive stomach before starting HRT, make sure you don't have another stomach problem, such as ulcers or polyps. Check your other medications and check for food allergy.

Leg cramps: There are many causes for leg cramps that can coincide with your hormone therapy. Adding more calcium to your diet and increasing your fluid intake should be the first line of attack. Adding magnesium to your diet though a dietary supplement may help. Sometimes, increasing your estrogen dose will reduce the likelihood of cramps.

It is important to note that hormone replacement therapy is of far lower potency than traditional birth-control pills. As a result, many of the feared side effects and risks of the Pill are not an issue. In other words, if you had problems tolerating the birth-control pill, it does not necessarily follow that you will have problems with estrogen replacement therapy.

In fact, low-dose oral contraceptives are often a good choice for women who need early replacement therapy as well as birth control. They are also particularly helpful for irregular bleeding that occurs in the perimenopause.

Other estrogen-related changes include:
- Changes in the shape of the eye that can make it difficult to wear contact lenses.
- Vaginal bleeding. May be a consequence of cyclic therapy or a side effect when occurring at the same time as the therapy.
- Gallstones. Some studies do show an increased incidence of gallstones, related to duration of hormone use.

As it turned out, Shawna had not yet tried very low dosages of some preparations. We placed her on a low dose of Estrace, 0.5mg every other day, which we later increased to five times per week. I also suggested she take vitamin E, while restricting her caffeine. Six months into her therapy, we find Shawna in great spirits with very occasional, tolerable breast sensitivity. We advised low-dose ibuprofen or similar anti-inflammatory agents to eliminate that symptom as needed. Because her dosage is lower than the recommended amount, I will evaluate her with regard to bone-density maintenance in approximately 18 months to two years. Her current therapy is a compromise to give her some of the benefits with fewer side effects.

Side Effects Fixers

• • •

The table on the next page summarizes the most common side effects, and some of the common fixes that can be tried to eliminate them. Your doctor should work with you to try to eliminate the side effects, and to figure out which fix works best for you.

Drug Interactions

Your doctors should know all the medications you are taking, as they may interact with your hormone therapy. The "side effects" caused by these interactions may not be obvious, nor have outcomes

Side Effect	Fix 1	Fix 2	Fix 3	Fix 4
Bloating	Lower salt intake.	Take a mild diuretic.	Lower the progestin dose.	Change the progestin type.
Weight gain	Modify diet.	Exercise designed to burn calories and fat as well as increase the metabolic rate.	Keep a food diary.	Join a weight-loss program.
Breast tenderness	Lower salt.	Lower estrogen.	Change the type or dose of progestin you're taking.	Cut down or eliminate caffeine.
Headaches	Lower your salt intake.	Change the type or dose of estrogen or progestin.	Change to a continuous schedule, if on cyclic.	Consider a non-oral estrogen regimen such as a patch.
Depression	Change from continuous to cyclic progestin or vice versa. (Note if the relationship is to the progestin or the estrogen.)	Take a hormone holiday, and see if it is in fact the cause.	Measure your hormone levels to see if they are adequate.	If you're on birth-control pills, try another with decreased progesterone/androgen effects.
Nausea	Take the tablets at bedtime, and/or with meals.	Try a non-oral product, such as a patch or gel.	Make sure you don't have another stomach problem.	Check your other medications and check for food allergy.
Leg cramps	Add more calcium to your diet.	Increase fluids.	Increase estrogen dose.	Add magnesium to your diet.

that you would expect. For example, a woman who takes a cholesterol-binding product at the same time as her estrogen supplement may deactivate all or part of the estrogen's potency. These two medications should be taken at least two hours apart to maintain effectiveness; I recommend taking one in the morning, and the other in the evening, if possible.

There are interactions with testosterone and other hormones as well. If the woman is using birth-control pills, the test must be drawn during the "off" week, days 1 through 5, or you can get very misleading results.

Sometimes the only way to be sure is to attempt a cautious and carefully administered "trial program" of hormone treatment and see if a woman's body responds positively. It may be helpful to use a screening and monitoring journal, such as the one in Appendix C.

Contraindications

Women may be advised *not* to use estrogen if they have the following conditions. These risks may be relative, and should be weighed against other risks and benefits.

- Breast cancer
- Abnormal uterine bleeding of unknown cause
- Extremely high triglyceride level
- A history of blood clots. If naturally occurring, you should be screened for clotting factors. If this is due to an accident or surgery, it does not present the same risks. You may have to avoid oral estrogens, for example, but be able to use other forms of estrogen such as transdermal patches or creams.
- History of severe liver disease. Because oral estrogens are metabolized by the liver, if liver enzymes test at normal, hormone replacement therapy may be okay. If not, non-oral estrogens may be used.

Cigarette smokers should quit while starting replacement therapy. Smoking lowers estrogen levels and the effectiveness of estrogen, and causes a multitude of serious health problems. It is not a contraindication in itself (as it is with birth-control pills), but it is counterproductive. Estrogen still helps the heart, and thus may actually be of particular benefit to smokers.

The Gospel Truth—SIDE EFFECTS: The Good, the Bad, and the Ugly

• • •

1. Possible negative side effects to hormone treatment include breast tenderness, vaginal bleeding, stomach upset, changes in skin pigmentation, weight gain, fluid retention, allergies and headache, depression, acne, headaches, PMS, fibroid enlargement, and irregular bleeding. Side effects from complications include nausea, gallstones, and dizziness.

2. Often, the side effects are not considered medically "serious," but they are serious in that they may stop women from taking their treatment.

3. Positive side effects include: suppression of endometriosis; improved sex drive; control of abnormal bleeding; improved mood, improved elasticity and resilience of vaginal tissues; improved libido and sexual performance; control of hot flashes, improved quality of sleep; better skin, hair, and nails; decrease in musculoskeletal aches and pains; improved mental functioning.

4. Often, the dosage of a hormone can determine whether it causes a condition, such as headaches, or improves it.

5. Women should consider the following conditions to be potential relative contraindications for estrogen: breast cancer, very high triglyceride level, history of blood clots, history of serious liver disease. Abnormal uterine bleeding of unknown cause is an absolute contraindication and should be examined immediately. Also, smokers should quit before taking estrogen.

15

SPECIAL CASES
Chemotherapy, Radiation, Surgery, Cancer Treatment, and Postpartum Depression

●　　●　　●

Vera, a 28-year-old single flight attendant with no children, who had radiation treatment for Hodgkin's disease, told me:

"I have hot flashes nearly all the time. Sometimes I can have them 20 times in an hour. It's literally impossible to think or work. I sweat like a stuck pig and my face turns beet red. I'm tired of people asking me if I'm all right. I had Hodgkin's disease last year and had radiation treatment. I still had periods for a while, then they stopped in the middle of therapy and my cancer specialist says I'm menopausal now. What does that mean? Is it permanent?"

Vera unfortunately had to fight cancer early in her life, and the depression of her natural hormone production created an artificially early menopause. Sometimes such artificially induced menopause can be temporary, but many times, it is permanent. It depends upon whether the woman's ovaries and egg follicles are only stressed by the therapy or permanently damaged. The intensity of menopause symptoms in young women can be quite severe when induced artificially. Artificial menopause comes with the same symptoms as natural menopause and the same physiological problems, such as the risk of osteoporosis and the acceleration of heart disease. Because the number of years of hormone deficiency may be more than doubled, it is important to treat early.

We gave Vera cyclic hormone replacement (Premarin at a dose of 0.9mg/daily, with 12 days a month of Provera at 0.5mg), which causes regular monthly bleeding. This was important to her, because it reinforced her feeling of normalcy. Her symptoms improved almost immediately. At 12 weeks, she sleeps through the night and is back to work. Unfortunately, it is unlikely she will ever be fertile. Hormone-induced cyclic bleeding isn't the same as your regular period; it doesn't have anything to do with ovulation. So far, Vera remains free of disease, but continues to undergo diligent monitoring. She will watch for more than one period a month on the chance that her hormone function returns. When acute estrogen loss occurs after severe stress, rather than surgery or menopause, it *can* rebound.

Tiffany is a divorced 38-year-old accountant with a history of endometriosis. Her uterus and right ovary were removed approximately four years ago. She told me:

"I haven't been the same since my hysterectomy. I just don't feel right. I find myself frequently depressed, moody, and I have these strange aches and pains in my bones and joints. I have a headache at least several times a week and sometimes it puts me to bed. Sex drive? What sex drive? I have no feelings even though I get along with my boyfriend just fine—luckily he's patient and I have sex to please him, but I might as well not be there. Help me, please!"

Any kind of major reproductive surgery disrupts the production and distribution of normal hormones. This type of artificially induced menopause is often called "surgical menopause." About 25 percent of American women will experience a surgical menopause and the subsequent acute, severe drop in hormones. The drop in estradiol, testosterone, and DHEA is approximately equal to the natural drop of menopause; the drop in estrone and androstenedione is actually greater from surgical menopause than natural. When the ovaries are removed entirely or substantially, it is like being cut off from hormones "cold turkey." This makes it more difficult than natural change of life. Many women describe it as the bottom dropping out of their lives.

When one or both ovaries are left behind, the changes may occur more slowly, but they will occur. Sometimes, the ovaries are in "shock" and recover later, meaning you might have symptoms for days or weeks immediately after the surgery which then resolve themselves. However, within two years, it is common to experience outright, permanent deficiency. This comes as a surprise not only to patients but also to many doctors; faced with a young woman who has at least one ovary, doctors often overlook the possibility of deficiency.

Removal of the ovaries also interferes with testosterone levels and lowers your sex drive. In this case your doctor should consider testosterone replacement earlier than with natural menopause.

Lupron, a drug sometimes prescribed for endometriosis, causes artificial, temporary menopause, and may also require hormone replacement therapy. This is sometimes called "add-back therapy."

Let's return to Tiffany, the woman with a history of endometriosis. She was placed on an estrogen/progesterone continuous regimen with testosterone. After 16 weeks of therapy, her sex drive has returned, although not totally to presurgery levels. Her other symptoms have subsided. We chose to continue progesterone even though her uterus was removed because it may help suppress any remaining remnants of endometriosis.

Hysterectomy

There is so much confusion and controversy regarding hysterectomy that we need to talk about how to determine when it is right for a woman and when it might not be.

Katrina, a patient with fibroids (benign muscle growths of the uterus) who came to me for a second opinion regarding hysterectomy, is an example of that confusion. She was 48 years old and did not feel she was menopausal. She had developed progressively heavier bleeding over a two-year period, with increased frequency and clotting. Her doctor detected several fibroids and concluded that they were the cause of her bleeding. She recommended hysterectomy to stop the bleeding.

This was not an unreasonable guess. Abnormal bleeding can be caused by many benign conditions, including fibroids, ovarian cysts, adenoymosis (a problem with uterine muscle), infections, and polyps, as well as cancer of any of the gynecological organs, particularly uterine and cervical cancer. However, abnormal bleeding is also one of the most common symptoms of menopause! This can be a too heavy or a too light period, bleeding between periods, increase in clots, periods closer together or farther apart. These symptoms may occur individually or in any combination of the above.

Confirming my suspicion, I found a significant hormone imbalance in Katrina's blood tests. We decided to attempt a trial of hormone replacement to control the bleeding. Over two months of therapy, the problem progressively improved and became tolerable. We measured the fibroids to be sure they were stable in size, and not suspicious in appearance. A biopsy of the uterine lining was done as well to detect any early cancer or precancerous change of the inside of the uterus. An iron supplement to her diet helped solve a slight anemia we had also detected in her blood tests. Katrina continues to do well two years later and has avoided a hysterectomy for now.

This approach is definitely worth a try if your symptoms are not too severe. Sometimes it proves to be a short-term solution, with the problem recurring later, but in other cases the abnormal bleeding never returns.

Of course, there are circumstances in which hysterectomy must be considered. If you have a precancerous or cancerous condition, a hysterectomy—as early as possible—is a lifesaving operation. Another condition that may require hysterectomy is a prolapsed (fallen) uterus. This typically occurs after childbirth or other stresses, such as chronic complications from lung disease, when the uterus loses its support structure and descends into the vagina. (It cannot fall completely out, because of its connections with internal structures.) The non-surgical approach is to use support devices called pessaries, which are inserted somewhat like a diaphragm. They come in various shapes and sizes, and are usually made of silicone. If you are *not* in good health or don't want surgery under any circumstances, then a pessary may be the best choice for you. However, if you are healthy, uterine prolapse should be fixed surgically by any of several procedures. Most involve removal of the uterus and restructuring of the support ligaments. If the problem is not taken care of early, when surgery is an option, it may progress and cause further discomfort for you at a time in your life when your health makes it difficult to consider a surgical repair. This problem can run in families with a history of weak connective tissue, so knowing your family history is helpful.

Another legitimate reason to consider hysterectomy or other surgical options is when bleeding is severe and doesn't respond to conservative approaches such as hormones, birth-control pills, or "D&C" (dilation and curettage, a surgical removal of the lining of the uterus). When bleeding causes frequent disruption of your life, as well as anemia, fatigue, insomnia, and headaches—in short, whenever your quality of life is suffering—this may outweigh the risks of the surgical alternatives. Some women may be candidates for uterine ablation, an option short of hysterectomy that involves cauterization of the lining of the uterus so it no longer develops and cannot shed as bleeding.

Pain resulting from scar tissue, endometriosis, or other causes should first be treated medically or with hormones, but if these fail, surgery may ultimately be the best choice. It is just as harmful to avoid a needed surgical procedure as it is to have an unnecessary one.

Hysterectomy may also be the last chance to control the growth and symptoms of fibroids as well, especially if they are multiple and growing fast. Many women who still want to have children opt for a myomectomy, the removal of the fibroid tumors that leaves the uterus and ovaries intact. The risk is that this leaves the door open for fibroids to return, which may require another surgery of either type. In certain cases, the fibroids can be "embolized," which means putting substances through a catheter into the fibroid's blood supply to interrupt the blood flow. This causes the tumor to decay and shrink. Postoperatively, this can be quite painful for a period of time.

If you do have a hysterectomy, note that recuperation is quicker and hospitalization is shorter when the procedure is done vaginally than by abdominal incision. Unfortunately, the vaginal hysterectomy is not always possible when the uterus is too large, when there is dense scar tissue present, or if cancer is a concern.

The abdominal surgery uses either a "bikini" style incision—low, transverse across the abdomen—or, less commonly, a vertical one. Muscles are only cut if exceptional exposure is required, as with some cancer surgeries or difficult procedures.

The decision to remove or spare the ovaries is a separate one. This depends on your age, the surgical technique used, the ovaries' position, and whether or not the ovaries are normal. Removal of the ovaries is not necessarily required just because you are having a hysterectomy, but it may make sense.

Treating your hormone imbalance is very important if you're having a hysterectomy. There are few things worse than a successful surgical procedure followed by severe depression and emotional stress due to a sudden hormone drop. You should be given a shot of estrogen in the recovery room, or put on a patch right away, to avoid the consequences of a sudden drop in hormone levels.

A hysterectomy can be a great choice or a horrible alternative depending on the circumstance. An unnecessary surgery is never the right thing, but a necessary one can be lifesaving.

Zoe is a married, 49-year-old receptionist who completed treatment for early-stage cancer of the left breast with a lumpectomy and radiation. She had been on tamoxifen therapy for about a year when she told me:

"I'm here because I'm having a lot of side effects from my treatment. My vagina is paper-thin and bleeds from tearing. I have no desire to have sex, which aggravates an already difficult time for my husband; he still is not coping with my breast cancer very well. I don't dare interrupt my treatment and risk getting cancer again, but I'm having trouble. I'm very depressed, even though I have survived the treatment and my prognosis is good. I'm still suffering as though my case was very bad. I feel guilty for feeling this way when I should be relieved. Is there anything I can do for myself?"

Tamoxifen is a commonly used chemotherapeutic agent for breast cancer. It is effective even though it is itself a *weak* estrogen. It may seem strange to some that a strong estrogen may increase breast-cancer risk, while a weak one such as tamoxifen may be used to reduce it. However, tamoxifen works by blocking estrogen receptors in the breast and other tissues, preventing stimulation of the receptor and theoretically blocking changes leading to breast disease. In a prevention trial using women without breast cancer, but a strong risk factor profile, tamoxifen appears to be useful as a protection as well as a treatment. Unfortunately, this may present a double whammy. Women lose their hormones at about this age, and we are now exacerbating the symptoms of deficiency further with the tamoxifen therapy. This can create further trauma woven into an already stressful time.

Women who cannot take estrogen, or who may only take lower doses, may have problems controlling certain menopause symptoms. Sometimes if hot flashes are severe, higher-dose progesterone can be used to control them. Megace®, a type of progesterone, is used in 20–40mg/daily doses. Dosages of 800–1000 IU of vitamin E can improve or arrest hot flashes. Small amounts of locally applied estrogen creams and vaginal moisturizers can help dryness and aid in improving intercourse comfort. Testosterone can help on occasion, but is not effective in many cases for women in the absence of estrogen. Testosterone's effects are not fully known in this circumstance.

The easiest thing about Zoe's case was her depression. There are a number of effective antidepressants for short- or long-term treatment of depression and insomnia in women who are not candidates for estrogen. The antidepressants are not all alike—one may be terrible for you, while another may work wonderfully. They also take patience, as some of the benefits may take six weeks to be noticeable. I know a lot of women prefer taking over-the-counter supplements such as St. John's wort, but are fearful of traditional antidepressant medications. However, you have to approach both with caution, and both can play a role in improving symptoms. We'll discuss some of these over-the-counter products in detail in the next chapter.

Finally, though you might think that a woman with breast cancer should never take estrogen replacement therapy, in fact it is still an option. You have to look carefully at the severity of symptoms, the benefit expected, and the woman's particular tumor grade, cancer-cell differentiation, lymph-node status, receptors, and patient profile. We treat many breast-cancer survivors when the severity of symptoms and disturbance of their quality of life outweighs the small potential risk. Most women survive breast cancer (96 percent live at least five years and 71 percent survive at least 10 years) and have the desire to prevent osteoporosis and heart disease as well as receive any other estrogen benefits.

Back to Zoe, the receptionist who is taking tamoxifen and suffering from vaginal tearing: She and I decided together to use a small amount of local estrogen cream, ¼ of an applicator, three to four times a week, along with a vaginal moisturizer. We are evaluating her bone density to determine her osteoporosis profile. A low-dose antidepressant improved her sleep and her mood.

Four months after starting therapy, Zoe is seeing a 50 to 70 percent improvement. Her sex drive is not where she'd like it to be, but comfort during sex has returned. We are trying additional testosterone to help with her sex drive and will slowly adjust the dosage over a period of time. We will continue to monitor her condition as it changes and consider oral replacement of estrogen at a later date. Zoe's bone density will be reevaluated in 18 months; a single value of bone density is not as meaningful as a comparison between two values, since the *rate* of bone loss is the most important factor. It is critically important to monitor every woman's experience with hormones, because each will be unique and changing at unpredictable intervals. Some will need monthly adjustments. Some will go years before a change is required.

Bonnie, a 35-year-old architect and new mother, came into the office about six weeks after having her first child. She had a normal, uneventful vaginal delivery.

"I feel as though I am in a dark hole and can't pull myself out," Bonnie said. "I just had a baby and I should be happy, but I'm so sad I don't even want to pick up my own child. I feel despondent and isolated, and I know

no one in my family even understands how I feel. I don't want to go any-
where. I don't want to do anything, and I have no energy whatsoever. I am
afraid that I may hurt my baby, and I just don't care."

Recall that our hormone problems are due primarily to *changes*
in hormone levels, rather than to any absolute level. At different
times in your life, different hormone levels may be appropriate
and healthy, but sometimes the transition from one level to another may cause problems, especially if the change is radical. For
example, hormones surge during pregnancy, putting higher-than-
normal levels of estrogen into circulation in the body until delivery. Different women respond differently to the pregnancy
hormone changes. Some feel fabulous and well balanced while
pregnant and claim they've never felt better in their lives. Other
women are miserable from conception to delivery. So it is with the
radical drop in hormones, particularly estrogen, after delivery,
which typically causes a temporary lowering of mood—you may
have heard it called "the baby blues." In some women, the drop
and/or their response to their drop is particularly severe and
leads to postpartum depression that can be devastating, even life-
threatening. Hormonal treatment and antidepressant therapy,
along with psychological support, succeed when intervention is
prompt.

There is some evidence that women who suffer from postpartum depression may also suffer from depression not related to
pregnancy, or from manic-depression (unipolar and bipolar disorders). There seems to be further evidence that women who suffer
postpartum depression suffer a risk of relapse after another birth.
Some doctors suggest screening all women for depression after
birth, instead of waiting for the new mother to report it. Many
women are reluctant to report depression during what should be a
happy time because it makes them feel abnormal.

Postpartum psychosis is a more extreme disorder that may be
a mania, or may be bipolar; women with this psychosis often report hallucinations and delusions. It acts quickly and is so drastic
in its effect it requires immediate medical attention. Patients suffering from postpartum psychosis or severe postpartum depres-

sion often report suicidal or even homicidal tendencies. These patients may need complex pharmacological interventions in order to survive.

Generally, any woman who feels even mildly depressed, or who feels ambivalent or negative toward the new baby, for more than two weeks past childbirth should see a doctor. Postpartum depression and postpartum psychosis usually exhibit within a week or two of giving birth, although postpartum depression *may* take as long as three months to show symptoms. Women and their health-care providers should be wary of depression for up to a year after giving birth. Lack of sleep and the stress of caring for a new baby can cause any woman to feel tired or run down; this needs to be distinguished from true depression. A professional's opinion will be necessary, and ongoing follow-up as well.

Bonnie went through complete psychological and medical evaluations, which confirmed postpartum depression. I prescribed oral contraceptives, which helped balance her hormonal profile while her body was recovering, and a mild antidepressant. At her 12-week check, she was doing substantially better. She was able to take care of her baby, and relate to her family more positively. She will be monitored carefully until complete recovery, because relapses can occur. She and her family were cautioned that she is at risk for recurrence after another pregnancy.

The Gospel Truth—SPECIAL CASES: Chemotherapy, radiation, surgery, cancer treatment, and postpartum depression

• • •

1. Artificially induced menopause, such as that caused by treatments for certain cancers, surgery, and other causes, can result in more severe symptoms and physiological risks than regular menopause.
2. Removal of the uterus and ovaries can cause a "cold turkey" withdrawal of hormones with more severe symptoms than the natural change of life. Testosterone loss in this case (and in item 1 above) is also more pronounced.

3. Tamoxifen is a commonly used chemotherapeutic agent for breast cancer, and has been shown to have some of the positive effects of estrogen. Other effects of estrogen depletion may seem more severe or exacerbated in the face of tamoxifen use.
4. Antidepressants can be useful for treatment of estrogen-deficiency depression and sleep deprivation, with or without hormone replacement.
5. Hormones can be helpful in treating postpartum depression.

16

ALTERNATIVE MEDICINE
"I Prefer Not to Take Traditional Estrogen."

● ● ●

Jolene is a 54-year-old single businesswoman who came into my office with a large bag of herbal products, sat down, and threw her hands into the air, and said in exasperation.

"Look at all of these. I talk to my friends who know all about herbs and natural remedies, and this is what they tell me to take. I've seen herbal healers, holistic doctors, traditional doctors, and I've read a ton of magazine articles, and it doesn't make a difference at all. No matter what I take, I'm still miserable. I might as well try hormones."

I looked over the heap of "natural" and herbal remedies Jolene had dumped on my desk. The problem wasn't what she was taking; it was that she didn't really know what they were good for or how to use them properly. Worse, she would switch on and off—taking "megadoses" at times to try to quickly rid herself of a symptom. She complained of stomachaches, hot flashes, skin rashes, and nausea. Not only that, but a careful history revealed she was a highly allergic individual. She had suffered from asthma, skin sensitivities to detergents, and intermittent hives for most of her life. Her family history was very strong for allergy problems, which may have been contributing to her stomachaches, given the large number of pills she was taking.

Jolene is not alone. Estimates of the sale of herbal, botanical remedies, and other "nutritional" supplements, vary from about $1.5 billion a year to over $12 billion! There may be as many as

60 million Americans using some form of herbal supplement or remedy. While many of us are no doubt looking for lower-risk, more "natural" treatments to improve our general health, there are a large number of modern-day Ponce de Leóns, looking for that Fountain of Herbal Youth. But Jolene illustrates the fact that natural products can do more harm than good. Although they can be perfectly safe and well tolerated by most people, for a person with allergies to plants and plant extracts, they can be a source of unexpected side effects and ultimately, a failed therapeutic approach.

In addition, most of the therapies that are non-hormonal are aimed at relieving symptoms as opposed to treating the underlying condition. For example, one of the main symptoms for which people seek relief is the hot flash. Avoiding exacerbating factors such as heat, stress, and spicy food can decrease hot-flash incidents, and vitamin E can sometimes help suppress them. Many other symptoms can be covered up by tranquilizers, which do nothing to change your physiology but see to it that you don't care! Of all the options, tranquilizers are probably my least favorite alternative.

Elizabeth, another patient, had a story quite different from Jolene's. A 47-year-old high-school counselor, Elizabeth told me she had tried as many as 10 hormone replacement regimens with no relief.

"I don't know what I'm going to do. I've tried everything you doctors have thrown at me, and none of it works. I can't sleep, and I'm so tired at the end of the day, I can barely stay awake. It's not fair to the students I have to work with. Sometimes, I find myself drifting off in the middle of a counseling session. The fatigue is so intense, I just go home in the evening and crash on the couch. I don't want any more hormones. What about herbal remedies?"

Natural versus Synthetic

Many people are attracted to natural, as opposed to synthetic, substances in their health-care regimens. This seems to be rooted in a socialized belief that all medicine is bad, and natural body processes are meant to continue no matter how uncomfortable.

But what is natural? Is natural necessarily good? Despite popular sentiment, natural does not always equal good or safe, and synthetic does not always equal bad. After all, as we've pointed out, cancer-causing tobacco is natural, while many lifesaving medicines are completely synthetic. Forget the black-and-white scenario when it comes to hormones.

Let's define the terms to help us understand them:

- Synthetic substances are those that are chemically derived without a natural source.
- Natural substances are extracted from plants and animal products. They may or may not be refined.

Regulated products that are available by prescription can be naturally occurring substances that have been processed or refined; or they may be synthetic substances; or a mix of synthetic ingredients and natural.

Likewise, over-the-counter substances may be natural or synthetic. Typically, they are unregulated or loosely regulated. This does not necessarily mean they are of poor quality—it means simply that the industry doesn't have agreed-upon and mandated standards. Some manufacturers produce excellent products and some do not.

Natural substances have not been proven to be more effective in any way than artificially derived substances, and the risks of each still need to be studied. If you are one of those people who takes psychological comfort in using a "natural" substance, you should realize that many naturally occurring substances are actually quite difficult for the body to assimilate, and can be, in fact, lethal! Also note that "natural" hormones are not necessarily in the form found in the body.

That said, the following substances may be useful as alternatives to HRT treatments or as adjuncts to relieve menopausal symptoms. As part of a blended regimen they may allow you to use a lower dose of estrogen. Both natural and synthetic treatments may be given as injections, creams, patches, pills, and other applications.

VITAMINS, MINERALS, AND NUTRIENTS

Vitamin E

This vitamin has been a successful alternative in treating the temperature disturbances of hot flashes and night sweats. It also may be useful for associated breast pain found in fibrocystic breast disease and in other low-estrogen conditions. Vitamin E is a low-risk supplement and has antioxidant effects as well. (That is, it lowers the rate of oxidation of cells in your body tissues, thus reducing the chances of cancerous change.)

The most common suggested dosage is 800–1,200 IU daily. Caution: More is not better! At high doses, vitamin E has some anti-blood-clotting activity.

Most doctors and researchers can at least agree that vitamin E is an antioxidant and helps to prevent coronary artery disease. While it hasn't been proven definitively to relieve menopause symptoms, it may help some women, and it does not do any harm.

Lecithin

Lecithin acts as an emulsifier for vitamin E, which means it helps the body dissolve and absorb vitamin E. It is an essential substance in the body and occurs naturally in the cell membranes. It may protect against cardiovascular disease and is thought to be beneficial to the brain and liver. The usual dose is 200–500 mg/day.

Vitamins B5 and B6

Although all the B vitamins are helpful, B5 and B6 in particular are thought to minimize water retention, ease various symptoms, and may help reduce the effects of stress. Estrogen may increase the need for vitamin B6 in the body because it seems to interfere with the metabolization of related chemicals, but this is still controversial and has not been proven. (Women on birth-control pills occasionally have especially low levels of B vitamins.) It should be noted that high doses of B6 (more than 100mg/day) are associated with the risk of neurological problems in the form of nerve damage. Symptoms are numbness or tingling. The recommended doses are 1.5–100mg/day for B6, and 100mg/day for B5.

Vitamin C

Vitamin C helps to reduce hot flashes in some women. Its potency increases when it is taken in conjunction with a bioflavinoid, such as Hesperidin. Vitamin C also acts as an antioxidant, and it is critical for bone health. It is associated with a lower risk for cancer, heart disease, and stroke. A dose of 500mg a day will do, and can be found in many foods.

Vitamin A

Vitamin A has many health benefits, some of which are of particular interest to menopausal women and women on hormone therapy. Dietary vitamin A (as opposed to that taken in supplements) has been demonstrated to provide immune-boosting effects with various cancers. Beta-carotene, which converts to vitamin A in the body, has been linked to lowered risk for cardiovascular disease. On the other hand, some studies have linked excessively high vitamin A intake to an increased risk for osteoporosis, and others have linked beta-carotene to increased risk for cancer.[22] Vitamin A may be taken at 3,300–4,000 I.U./day OR beta-carotene may be substituted at up to 10,000 I.U./day.

Folic Acid

Although it does not directly relate to menopause, folic acid can work in combination with estrogen to make significant improvements to a woman's health, including reducing cardiovascular disease. (For younger women its most essential benefit is in preventing potential birth defects.) Additionally, folic acid has been linked to reduced risk of colon cancer. The recommended dose of folic acid is 400mcg (micrograms) per day, which can easily be reached with most multivitamin supplements. Check the label.

Chromium—One to Avoid

• • •

The mineral chromium increases metabolism, which makes it a common ingredient in over-the-counter, "natural" diet pills. Since weight gain is a common symptom of menopause, some women may take chromium to keep their weight down. Its usefulness has not been established, however, and it may have side effects. Generally, I recommend diet and exercise over supplements for weight control, even if the supplements are "natural."

Phytoestrogens (Plant-Based Estrogens)

Phytoestrogens are naturally occurring plant estrogens that can help to supplement a woman's estrogen production, especially early in perimenopause, or when a woman's symptoms are not too severe. It is important to note that phytoestrogens are still an estrogen source; they provide the same benefits but also many of the same potential side effects and risks of estrogen therapy.

However, preliminary studies do suggest that plant estrogens are less likely to trigger breast cancer.[23] They may also have protective benefits for the heart and bones as well.

The different types of plant estrogens are as follows:

Lignans	Found in almost all cereal grains and vegetables, with highest concentrations in the oilseeds (e.g., flaxseed)
Coumestans	Found in sunflower seeds, red clover, and bean sprouts
Isoflavones	Most commonly found in legumes, with large concentrations in soybeans

Soy

The regimen with the strongest evidence for relieving menopausal symptoms is a low-fat diet with increased soy protein, and regular exercise. Although no definitive answers exist, studies suggest that soy helps alleviate hot flashes and other menopausal symptoms, osteoporosis, and heart disease, and may lower the risk of breast and uterine cancers.

Soy is available in many different products, making it somewhat easier to take than just raw beans for women who are "finicky" eaters, or have particular dietary requirements. Tofu, or soy curd, is bland by itself and has a texture that seems unusual to many Western palates. It may be used as a replacement or supplement for cottage or ricotta cheese or sour cream, as an ingredient in ice cream, or even as a thickener in certain soup recipes. Tofu essentially acquires the flavor of whatever it is mixed with, so it is adaptable into many recipes, and can be "masked" if desired. Additionally, soybeans may be eaten as green beans, roasted like peanuts, and enjoyed as soy sauce. (Those on low-sodium diets should use low-salt or "light" type soy sauce.) There are several brands of soy "milk," available at health-food stores and even grocery stores in some cities, that come in various flavors (i.e., chocolate, vanilla, and plain). While not necessarily milklike in taste, they are a good source of soy and soy protein (and may in some cases be substituted for milk for women who are lactose-intolerant).

The amount of isoflavone in various soy foods varies based on product source, formulation, and preparation. The estimated isoflavone content of various soy foods is as follows:

Food	Serving Size	Isoflavone Content
Tofu	4 oz	35–112mg
Miso soup	½ cup	40mg
Soy milk	1 cup	20–40mg
Texturized soy protein	4 oz	140mg
Roasted soy beans	4 oz	60–160mg
Green soy	4 oz	135mg

Soy is also available in supplement form, as tablets, capsules, or "protein powder." Some people are allergic to soy products. Large quantities of soy may cause gastrointestinal upset. Note that just because a product contains soy does not mean it contains soy *protein;* also, check the fat content—not all soy products are low in fat or fat-free. Soy milk and tofu may be high-fat and high-calorie products.

Flaxseed

Flaxseed has been associated with decreased vaginal symptoms and hot flashes in menopausal women.

DHEA

DHEA and DHEAS (DHEA-sulfate) are steroids produced by the body's adrenal glands in diminishing quantities as we age; we experience the lowest DHEA levels in the year before we die. This has led many people to believe that adding DHEA-based substances to the diet would provide a "Fountain of Youth," or anti-aging effect.

Unfortunately, DHEA has not proven as effective as many first hoped, but there may be a future in it. Information is still scarce. The best long-term or short-term dosages, side effects, and risks are still unknown. There have been some reports of liver damage with large doses, and of "androgenic" effects; that is, DHEA may make you more "manly" or manlike. For some reason women show a more dramatic increase of testosterone when taking DHEA than men. DHEA also appears to increase low-density lipoproteins, or LDLs (bad cholesterol), in women and can cause acne and hair loss.

Although I generally recommend against DHEA right now, I include it for discussion here because its use is fairly widespread, and it is important to weigh the benefits against the negative effect.

HERBS

Herbal or botanical products commonly used in treating menopause include: angelica, chamomile, clover, cohosh, damiana, dandelion, dong quai, evening primrose, kava kava, licorice, nettle, red raspberry, saw palmetto, uva ursi, and valerian root.

Note that just because some people use these substances and claim benefits, doesn't mean they are effective. Most are relatively harmless when properly taken, although they can cause reactions in people who are allergic to them. Some may be more toxic and dangerous in large quantities than others. Many have established benefits, while others, such as dandelion and red raspberry, seem to have no medical value at all. In some cases, such as with dong quai, there is no research or medical literature supporting its use.

Many over-the-counter herbal preparations may contain plant estrogens and alleviate your symptoms as a result of those low doses of estrogen. Other preparations may not contain these phytoestrogens, yet still treat related symptoms. The biggest problem with unregulated, over-the-counter treatments is that the concentration of active ingredients is not guaranteed. There's really no way to tell how much of the substance you're trying to take is actually *in* the supplement. Stick to well-known companies with reputations for delivering quality products. When tested, some herbal remedies were shown to contain *none* of the "active" ingredient! Reputable companies hold their own high standards in production.

Find a product that contains standardized extracts, so you know how much of the active ingredient you are getting, and in what form. The label should describe the percentage of extract, the full list of active ingredients, and the manufacturer. Beware of health-food stores and "herb shops" that sell items in poorly marked or handwritten containers. Don't forget that the federal government allows such "food" products to be sold as long as they have not been proved unsafe and make no health claims. That's why you'll often find ambiguous statements on their packages, such as "optimum natural benefits" or "heightens mental awareness"—well, caffeine "heightens mental awareness," and so do orange juice or a cold splash of water in the face! Rely on research and scientific studies rather than marketing slogans and advertising claims.

Another important fact many people may not realize is that while an individual herb may be safe, certain mixtures of herbs may not be. You can't just randomly throw them together. People accustomed to mixing their daily batch of vitamins may be mixing a dangerous cocktail if they do the same thing with herbs.

If you've decided to try a particular herbal remedy, follow the manufacturer's dosage recommendations. Don't go on and off the remedy; many herbal products act slowly, and will take time to produce an effect. Some could take several months to work at full efficiency. Don't take megadoses in the hopes of "jump-starting" the effect: Herbs that are safe or benign in small doses can trigger allergic reactions in larger doses, and possibly lead to severe complications, including death.

There is no data on long-term effects of continuous herbal therapies. They may turn out to be okay for long-term use, or it may turn out that herbs are safe in the short run, but not in the long run. For example, even some proponents of black cohosh recommend it for no more than six months at a time. If you're taking it for hot flashes, what do you do the other six months of the year?

If you are: (1) under a doctor's care for a chronic medical condition; (2) taking medication for an ongoing problem, or (3) pregnant or nursing, see your doctor before trying any herbal remedy. If you are healthy but seeking menopausal relief, talk it over with a health professional familiar with both herbs and your condition.

Some helpful herbal preparations:

Dong quai is a form of angelica often claimed to relieve cramps, hot flashes, vaginal dryness and other complaints. It has not been shown to cause growth of the lining of the uterus, nor to have effects on the vagina, but additional study is needed to better understand its benefits and risks. Some studies have shown dong quai to be no more helpful than placebo. Dong quai is contraindicated (that means you should avoid it) in instances of hemorrhagic disease, heavy periods, or pregnancy. It should not be used during menstruation. Dong quai elevates blood-sugar levels and should be avoided by diabetics. It also causes photosensitivity (exaggerated reaction of the skin to the sun).

Angelica itself interacts poorly with laxatives, aspirin, and antacids, and should be avoided by pregnant women and women with chronic problems with the gastrointestinal tract. Like dong quai, it may also cause photosensitivity (exaggerated reaction of the skin to the sun).

There are three types of *ginseng:* Siberian, American, and Chinese. It has been compared in studies with a placebo, and has definitely increased the psychological well-being of the women who took it. On the other hand, there have been some reports that ginseng can cause abnormal uterine bleeding, which has been equated with an estrogenic-like activity. Women with lung problems, rheumatic heart disease, or history of heart attack should avoid ginseng, because it increases blood pressure and adrenaline. It may also interfere with the blood-thinning effects of coumadin, an anticoagulant prescribed for certain heart and blood ailments. Ginseng may be linked with breast pain, vaginal bleeding, and insomnia.

Black cohosh, also called squaw vine, squawroot, or snakeroot. It is sometimes sold under the brand name Remifemin®, and is among the most popular of the over-the-counter menopause aids. Its claim to fame is it controls hot flashes. Black cohosh was used by Native Americans to relieve cramps and ease labor. As with most of the herbs mentioned here, there have been no large, well-designed studies to date, to actually prove benefit, although some smaller studies show some potential for treatment of hot flashes and improving vaginal tissue health. Black cohosh is not to be used by pregnant women or people with heart disease. It may cause nausea and vomiting if overdosed. Note: black cohosh and blue cohosh are not the same. Blue cohosh is more toxic and is not recommended.

Gingko biloba is an herb that has been touted for improving mental acuity and concentration. It is available in pill, powder, and tea forms, and is even added to sodas and candy bars commonly found in health stores. Its benefits and risks still require much study. It seems to have some of the mind-sharpening effects of caffeine or orange juice, and some of the blood-thinning activity associated with aspirin. It does not seem to be the "smart pill" some of its more vocal advocates claim it to be. There is some controversy over the gingko content of some supplements. The amount of extract, and whether that extract was derived from the full leaf of the plant may play some part in the product's potency.

St. John's wort has been touted as an "herbal Prozac" since the U.S. media discovered German and other European studies that found it to work as an antidepressant. However, as with prescription antidepressants, it can take weeks to have a noticeable effect and there are risks and side effects associated with it. As I've mentioned before, just because a drug is natural, doesn't mean it is safe. St. John's wort is known to cause photosensitivity, which may lead to quicker and more severe sunburn, especially in fair-complexioned people. It also interacts with other drugs, particularly the class of blood pressure medications called "MAO inhibitors"; do not mix the two. St. John's wort is usually sold as a standardized extract of hypericum because that is the chemical ingredient that is easiest to measure. (In other words, the bottle will say "Hypericum: 300mg" or something similar.) It should be noted that hypericum itself does not seem to be the active ingredient—researchers are still trying to isolate the ingredient in St. John's wort that alleviates depression. Therefore, while a St. John's wort product you buy may be standardized, there is no guarantee that it contains any of the active ingredient you are seeking.

Depression may be a sign of other health or mental problems; it should not be self-diagnosed, nor self-treated. A doctor can best diagnose and treat you if you are feeling "down." This does not rule out the use of natural substances, but with either, depression requires supervision.

Valerian root is often used as a sleep aid and tranquilizer, though there are no good scientific studies validating its efficacy. Valerian lowers blood pressure, and should be avoided by women taking blood pressure medication or anticoagulants.

Sage, raspberry, gotu kola, and *belladonna* have also been claimed to have positive health benefits with regard to menopause symptoms. *Licorice* and *licorice root* are thought to stimulate estrogen production. These substances are available variously as powders, teas, capsules, liquid extracts, and in their raw, unprocessed state. *Marigold ointment* is sold as a natural aid for vaginal itching. While I don't discourage my patients from taking these remedies within reason, I do not recommend them either, because their efficacy is not proven. They should be taken with your doctor's knowledge and supervision.

The Chinese herb *ma huang,* which is also known by its Western name, *ephedra,* is a popular caffeinelike substance often used for weight loss, and is sometimes found in diet powders. However, it has been associated with various complications, including death. Menopausal women looking to trim off some of the weight gain often associated with this phase of life would be better off with tried-and-true methods such as diet and exercise, no matter how difficult. Whatever your preference, you should consult your physician before beginning any serious weight-loss program.

In general, over-the-counter herbal preparations can be very helpful in the early stages of menopause, when the symptoms are not yet severe. As the symptoms increase in intensity, a woman will often find that these preparations are no longer enough and she will need to gradually shift to a doctor-prescribed treatment, which may also be natural.

Remember, if there is a reason you are avoiding estrogen, such as a personal history of breast cancer, or other contraindications, natural estrogen may not necessarily be any safer, and used to excess, could even be dangerous. A professional's guidance in these areas is imperative. If you still have your uterus, it must be protected with progesterone while on *any* estrogen.

If you do seek the guidance of alternative medical practitioners, such as chiropractors, acupuncturists, herbalists, homeopaths, osteopaths, and various Eastern and other cultural specialists, find out how knowledgeable they are about menopause, and make sure you keep your medical doctor informed about what you're doing. An alternative treatment may conflict with, oppose, or otherwise interact with a conventional medicine or treatment you are receiving. This is important, even if you suspect your doctor would not approve of alternative treatments. It is your right to seek them out. Just play it safe and inform all your health-care providers of everything you are taking and whether you are experiencing any side effects.

FOODS

Common foods are often overlooked in the search for health benefits *treatments*. Apples, cherries, pomegranates, flaxseed, alfalfa, barley, hops, oats, rice, wheat, legumes, peas, potatoes, sprouts, Mexican yams, fennel, garlic, parsley, and sesame seeds have all been reported to relieve menopause symptoms. Fish oils have been credited for reducing menopausal symptoms in Asian and Inuit women, as well as greatly lowering the risk of cardiovascular disease. They contain omega-3 fatty acids, which may act as a "blood thinner." Fish oils have been used as a potential breast cancer reduction treatment or preventative, and may decrease the risk of colon cancer.

Additional relief can be found from blackstrap molasses, broccoli, dandelion greens, kelp, salmon with bones, sardines, and low-fat yogurt, all of which contain calcium and may help prevent or slow osteoporosis.

On the other hand, avoiding certain foods can be as important as taking others. Dairy products, sugar, red meat, alcohol, caffeine, and spicy foods may contribute to hot flashes in some women.

It also seems that hypoglycemic women may have more pronounced menopause symptoms in general. It is important to check for both high and low blood-sugar levels, as well as thyroid dysfunction.

ANTIDEPRESSANTS

Antidepressants and tranquilizers are certainly not "alternative" medicine, in the sense that we use the word today, to mean natural or holistic. However, many women take these drugs as an "alternative" to estrogen to treat symptoms of menopause, with or without their doctor's understanding of what is really being treated.

Antidepressant therapy can certainly be used in conjunction with HRT or by itself to alleviate symptoms, but they should not be used to "cover up" symptoms without addressing the underlying conditions. Three well-known and often-used antidepressants are Prozac, Zoloft, and Paxil. All three of these are in the "serotonin-boosting family" of mood enhancing agents, which means they work by increasing the body's natural levels of serotonin. Although they don't control hot flashes per se, they can help control mood swings and depression, improve quality of sleep, and improve general well-being. It appears that low doses of these compounds can enhance the effectiveness of estrogen and therefore may lower the dose of estrogen you need to alleviate symptoms. There are many other excellent antidepressants that work on different chemical imbalances, such as Wellbutrin, which boosts norepinephrine, a substance in the body that functions as an energy enhancer. Again, a professional's guidance is imperative.

HRT can sometimes exacerbate the symptoms of other conditions. For example, estrogen may increase your fluid retention or, less commonly, asthma or migraine headache symptoms. It can also improve other conditions, such as migraine headaches (yes, it can make them better *or* worse!), and arthritic syndromes.

TRANQUILIZERS

Although tranquilizers can be useful in the short term for anxiety, stress, and other problems, they are not generally a good long-term option for several reasons: (1) their addictive nature; (2) their tendency to cause drowsiness and a mental fog; and (3) "hangover effect" (waking up the next morning feeling as though you have a hangover).

PROGESTERONE

This nonestrogen female hormone is also used to treat temperature disturbances, as well as provide some protection of bone. It is also useful in conjunction with estrogen when there is an endometriosis or uterine cancer history. The safety and/or efficacy of long-term progesterone in different forms is still not clear. It can also cause some very bothersome side effects, such as breast pain, bloating, moodiness, depression and irritability, headaches, abnormal bleeding, and oily skin, acne, and other skin disruptions.

Progesterone-only studies that have shown increased bone density have not been set up to eliminate outside factors. For example, the women in some of these studies were also on exercise regimens, calcium, vitamins, and minerals. Two-thirds of the women were on estrogen replacement, too. There continues to be debate on progesterone's ability to prevent osteoporosis, although it clearly provides relief from hot flashes when taken orally. The benefits of progesterone creams are not clear for this symptom.

Contrary to some beliefs, even though some progesterone supplements and creams are derived from wild yams, you cannot eat yams to supplement estrogen or progesterone. It just takes too many yams to make even a little bit of progesterone, which the body won't absorb!

Another choice for progesterone that is well absorbed is the intervaginal preparation Crinone gel. This is different from progesterone skin creams, because the vaginal tissue absorbs substances differently than skin does. It is effective and predictable. Crinone gel is a particularly good alternative for women who are intolerant to the other oral progesterones. The gel is a 4 percent solution that can be used in a continuous regimen, two times a week, or cyclically, every other day.

The CombiPatch combined estrogen/progesterone patch puts the hormones into a "matrix"—a sort of miniaturized, high-tech, time-release poultice—making it easier to absorb.

LOCAL CREAMS (ESTROGEN AND PROGESTERONE)

For women who have suffered from breast cancer, or are otherwise unable to take normal oral doses of estrogen, low-dose estrogen creams can be used to relieve vaginal dryness "locally" without the danger of cell stimulation.

Progesterone creams may alleviate some women's symptoms such as hot flashes, cycle irregularity, and even bone loss. Generally, I feel that the efficacy of progesterone in the absence of estrogen, regardless of the source, is somewhat overstated. We still don't have enough information about the risks and benefits of progesterone in its newer forms; studies have found both negative effects *and* breast-protective effects! Regardless of source, topical progesterone creams are poorly absorbed through the skin and unlike estrogen, require a large surface area to achieve any absorption.

If you are using a progesterone cream, do not assume it is protecting you against precancerous and cancerous uterine change; if you are taking estrogen as well, you must be monitored as though you are taking it alone (unopposed).

CALCIUM, FOSAMAX, AND OTHER BONE-BUILDERS

Since estrogen helps prevent osteoporosis, women who can't take estrogen (or choose not to) often need another form of treatment in order to maintain healthy bones. Calcium is an essential mineral that is available from many sources, including dairy products, green leafy vegetables, and certain seafood. Tums® (or any calcium carbonate–based supplement) is an inexpensive calcium source. If calcium carbonate causes gastrointestinal upset, try alternate sources such as citrate, gluconate, and lactate. Elemental calcium—which you may think of as calcium in its molecularly "pure" form—is the critical element in any calcium supplement. Finding a supplement with elemental calcium in the correct amount is the goal in finding the correct supplement for you. Calcium carbonate has the highest elemental calcium content, at 40 percent. Lactate has about 13 percent and gluconate about nine.

After the elemental calcium content, the next most important factor is the "dissolution" or absorption rate of the dose. The better calcium supplements have as much as 90 percent dissolution within an hour of taking the dose. Some of the generic calcium supplements available at your pharmacy or supermarket have dissolution rates of as little as 6 to 13 percent. It is important to read the label carefully, or to get a recommendation from a doctor or nutritionist, to assure yourself of taking a calcium supplement that will actually help.

Regardless of the supplement you take, you will often get better results if you split the dose; that is, don't take it all at once. This produces better absorption and metabolism of the dose by your body, and reduces the risk of stomach upset some people get if they take too much calcium. You might take half in the morning and half in the evening; taking a third with each meal might even be better, since calcium is absorbed better when taken with food (this can also help reduce any gastric upset).

Taking 1,200mg to 1,500mg daily should be sufficient. Don't

take more than 2,000mg/day. Larger doses have potential risks and show no increased benefit.

Along with magnesium, calcium may also help relieve nervousness and irritability.

Fosamax is a brand name for alendronate, a preparation of bisphosphonate that has been shown to inhibit osteoporosis. You have to take it on an empty stomach with a lot of water, and then remain upright for 30 minutes. The benefit is worth the trouble if osteoporosis is your problem. However, some women experience stomach upset too severe to continue taking it.

Other substances that may help the bones are vitamins C and D, and the minerals magnesium, boron, and phosphorus.

PLACEBO EFFECT

Strangely enough, in almost all double-blind studies, in which one group of patients receives a new treatment while the other receives a placebo (pill or regimen with no active ingredient), a certain number of patients will respond favorably to the placebo. This "placebo effect" happens with all forms of treatment, whether alternative or traditional, Western or Eastern, medicinal or herbal. In one recent study regarding baldness, 42 percent of the men taking a placebo reported increased scalp-hair growth, compared to 86 percent of the men taking the active medication! The placebo effect should never be used to dismiss a therapy outright, and in fact reminds us of the power of the mind and its importance in health. As we have said, if it works and causes no harm, why not?

LIFE ENHANCEMENTS

It is important to separate alternative medicine from alternative approaches such as exercise, behavioral treatment, and acupuncture that are "adjunct therapies." Changes in lifestyle or behavior can theoretically boost your body's self-healing ability. Their benefits are difficult to assess from patient to patient because of the difficulty of designing effective studies. But numerous studies show that exercise and behavioral treatments—such as relaxation techniques, paced respiration, yoga, acupuncture, and acupressure—

enhance the general health and well-being of the body, and if nothing else may help you better cope with your symptoms. This is always a goal, regardless of your decision on hormone intervention. It is cruel, however, to imply that if a woman faithfully exercises, watches her diet, and so on, she will be fine without hormones— she may not.

After reviewing with Jolene the effects and side effects of her multitude of herbal remedies, we decided to switch her off of natural compounds until her body cleared the effects, while monitoring her diet and environment for other potential side effect causes. After the clearing period, we initiated low-dose, synthetic-estrogen replacement, which arrested her hot flashes and improved her sleep. As a businesswoman, she no longer dreads leading client meetings for fear of drowning in a pool of sweat.

Elizabeth, the patient who had tried hormones without success and wanted an herbal remedy for her fatigue, was much tougher to figure out. Her hormone-screening tests were all normal. Because of her fatigue, we did a blood-sugar screen, thyroid evaluation, and check of her blood count to see if she was anemic. Since some forms of thyroid disease are difficult to detect and involve different processes, I also ordered a test of thyroid antibody levels. This reveals more unusual causes of thyroid problems, which may cause hot flashes and sweats. The test results indicated Elizabeth had high blood sugar (early diabetes) and a thyroid imbalance. We recommended a diabetic nutrition program, increased her exercise regimen, and supplemented her thyroid hormone. We also boosted soy in her diet. Elizabeth's fatigue improved dramatically after treatment, and she didn't require estrogen at all. To date, she has no increase in symptoms and is doing well.

The Gospel Truth—ALTERNATIVE MEDICINE: "I Prefer Not to Take Traditional Estrogen."

• • •

1. Synthetic substances are those that are chemically derived. Natural substances are extracted from plants and animal products found in nature.

2. Natural does not always equate to "good," just as synthetic does not always equate to "bad."

3. Although no other substance is a perfect substitute for estrogen, many substances may be useful to complement or replace estrogen in control of symptoms.

4. Vitamins, especially E, may help with menopause symptoms and offer an alternative treatment.

5. Phytoestrogens, which are naturally occurring plant estrogens, may help with menopause symptoms. However, it is important to remember that they are still estrogen and may have the same negative effects, including uterine and breast-cell stimulation.

6. Over-the-counter herbal remedies may be helpful in the early stages of menopause, but often become less helpful as the symptoms become more severe, or in the absence of professional guidance. Their quality is uneven.

7. Many foods and other environmental influences may increase or decrease the severity of menopause symptoms.

8. Many prescription medications may interact with the body in a way that may mask or exacerbate menopause symptoms. They may also interact with hormone replacement therapy in the same way.

9. Calcium, along with other new bone-building agents, is even more important to reduce the risk of osteoporosis for women who do not take estrogen.

10. The menopause *can* be managed successfully without estrogen for some women.

17

CULTURAL VARIATIONS, GENETICS, ENVIRONMENT
"My Mother Made Me Do It."

•   •   •

Akiko, a 68-year old Asian woman, was in my office for another reason when she confessed she was having trouble sleeping. She said:

"I haven't slept well for over 10 years, I've been coping with it, using over-the-counter products and a few folk remedies my mother taught me back in Japan. But lately, I wake up drenched in sweat. It is almost like I have been swimming. My skin is clammy, and the sheets are damp. I read a magazine article that said this could be due to lack of hormones. Can that be possible at my age? I finished menopause years ago, just after I moved to the U.S."

We don't know nearly enough about hormones, their replacement, and the importance of their sources; to compound our ignorance we are also often blind to cultural variations and differences in individual response. Although there is undoubtedly a genetic basis for the discrepancies, there is also a profoundly important environmental influence. This has been amply demonstrated by comparing the incidence of certain diseases among women in their homelands as compared to the U.S. These studies show that regardless of the rates of disease in their homelands, women tend to adjust to the disease rate of where they are now living. For example, the incidence of breast cancer among Asian women living in Asia is lower than that of Asian women who live in the United

States. In other words, environmental factors are just as critical as other factors, such as genetics.

That isn't to negate the importance of genetics. One recent Mayo Clinic study of white ethnic groups found significant differences in breast cancer risk based on country of descent. American women of Scandinavian descent were at the greatest risk, those of Irish heritage were at the lowest. The study also found that nationality affected the importance of family history with regard to risk. Strangely, the same Irish and Scandinavian nationalities both rated lowest among correlation to family history, while English, Welsh, Dutch, German, and other Europeans had stronger correlation.[24]

Many studies are attempting to determine which cultural behaviors decrease disease, such as diet, and can be used by anyone to improve their health, regardless of their original "home culture."

For example, the Inuit (Eskimo) diet, which is high in fish oils containing omega-3 fatty acids, protects against cardiovascular disease through various mechanisms. These include decreasing platelet aggregation, preventing cardiac arrhythmia, and reducing triglyceride levels, according to research conducted by Dr. Bruce Holub, a professor in the Department of Human Biology and Nutritional Science at Guelph (Ontario) University.[25]

The Japanese, who have a diet high in fish oils and soy, have only a quarter of the heart disease mortality reported by North Americans. In addition, Japanese women have a tenfold decrease in reported hot flashes, according to Dr. Gregory Burke, professor and vice chairman in the Department of Public Health Sciences at Wake Forest University in Winston-Salem, North Carolina.[26]

The environmental differences that contribute to these statistics may include nutrition, native pollution (or absence of it), exposure to toxins such as tobacco, alcohol, and radiation, changes in reproductive age, sexual habits, and stress levels.

In addition to knowing the genetic basis of disease, environmental influences, and the latest technical advances, health-care providers must grapple with understanding the emotional framework of a patient. This will affect the specific therapy used as well as health-care decision making in general. Social influences are very powerful and must be understood in order to penetrate a preexisting framework that may cause someone to avoid or sabotage treatment. Some women are brought up in families that encourage frequent positive experiences with medical care, focused on wellness and prevention, dental, eye, and medical checkups. Other families neglect regular health care and may even place it in a punitive role, creating fear and a mistrust of health-care services.

Cultural attitudes toward menopause, levels of education, and economic status are all significant in determining how a woman in menopause utilizes the health-care system (or not). Most well known are the differences between Japanese women living in Japan and American women. Japanese women reportedly experience the menopause much more positively, with many fewer symptoms, such as hot flashes, and are more accepting of the natural process.

However, what conclusions can we really draw from this report? The experience may well differ from culture to culture, country of origin, etc., but might not the reporting and documentation vary as well? The symptoms that are significant to a woman are those that bother *her* the most, not the physician. The standard well-known signs and symptoms may not include the woman's highest concerns, and she may not report others that don't disturb her.

Akiko was reluctant to take traditional therapy, but after evaluating her saliva and blood levels, in combination with her severe symptoms, it was clear that the effect of hormone deficiency was profound, and she was unlikely to get significant relief of her sleep disorder without some intervention. We custom-blended an estrogen/testosterone/progesterone cream at approximately 30 percent of the average replacement dose. She applied it at bedtime and almost immediately stopped waking up at 3 A.M., as had become her ritual. Her osteoporosis screening also revealed moderate loss of bone, which is consistent with several of her risk factors. We placed her on calcium-rich diet supplements at 1500mg/day, and weight-dependent exercise, along with the cream as discussed. We were able to demonstrate no further loss of bone after a 12-month interval. This treatment regimen was a compromise comfortable for Akiko; lower doses from natural sources helped arrest some of her more disturbing symptoms, and she could live with the treatment, with regard to side effects.

In conclusion, it is difficult to take anecdotal reports of non-American women having glorious and symptom-free menopause at face value. While there may indeed be dietary, cultural, genetic, and environmental conditions that improve one factor or another, the study and reporting of women's health issues in other countries needs improvement before conclusions may be drawn. And any lessening of menopause symptoms that may have been enjoyed by immigrant women in their home countries may be nullified by their new American lifestyles, or worse yet, their symptoms may be worse than the general population! These cultural and environmental factors require additional study before we can hope to understand and use them to improve the menopause experience for American women and their immigrant sisters.

The Gospel Truth—CULTURAL VARIATIONS, GENETICS, ENVIRONMENT: "My Mother Made Me Do It."

• • •

1. Ethnicity may affect how a woman's body reacts to menopause, as well as how the woman and her family feel about aging in general. The results may be due as much to environmental factors such as nutrition and psychological factors as they are to genetics.
2. Cultures with diets high in natural fish oils, soy products, and certain other foods seem to fare better in regards to the menopause experience. It is thought that some of these foods also help guard against cardiovascular disease.
3. Other factors, such as nutrition, environmental pollution, exposure to toxins such as tobacco, alcohol, pesticides, and radiation, changes in reproductive age, sexual habits, and stress levels, may also greatly affect responses to menopause.
4. Economics, spiritual beliefs, and religious practices may affect a woman's choice of health-care options and affect her success.
5. Education level is one of the single most important determinants of good health, even more so than economic level.

18

HUSBANDS, PARTNERS, AND FAMILY
No Woman Is an Island

•   •   •

Matthew, a 55-year-old aerospace executive, called me concerning his 45-year-old wife, Lela. She had been to my office for a routine checkup, and although I had questioned her about any menopausal symptoms, she said she was doing great.

Matthew had another perspective.

"If she knew I was calling you, she'd kill me, so don't tell her, please. I have to talk to you, I had to talk to someone, because things just aren't going very well. "

I told Matthew I'd be happy to talk with him, though I'd be unable to share any specifics about his wife's condition, since that's privileged information between a doctor and patient. I would certainly listen to his input, utilize that information to provide her with better care, and answer any general questions he might have. He told me they had been married for 12 years, and that over the last year or year and a half, she'd been getting up at 2 in the morning and wandering around the house because she couldn't get back to sleep. For the last few months, she had been extremely irritable and moody. She does have a high-pressure job in a printing business, but she had always been able to cope with her job stress before. She often "snaps his head off" when they're talking, without warning, or bursts into tears during a harmless commercial. Lela's coworkers had confided to Matthew that she's hard to work with, and may be endangering her job because of her erratic behavior.

They had a very healthy sex life up until a year or so ago, when it deteriorated substantially. "I love my wife," Matthew said, "but you have to help me help her, because I'm not sure how much more I can take."

This kind of case illustrates how a woman can be in a state of denial concerning her hormonal balance and the significant impact it may be having on her life. Sometimes women have gotten so used to feeling bad and putting up with it, they don't notice. As the old song says, "I've been down so long it looks like up to me."

Another reason some women ignore their symptoms is that they are so used to the caretaker role that they worry about everyone but themselves. Women are often also very tough physically; after all, they survive labor and childbirth on a regular basis, and effectively deal with physical limitations. Finally, the changes are often so subtle that the people around her are actually better able to define them than she is herself. No matter how well we know ourselves, the outside perspective of our family and friends provides valuable insight into our behavior and objective information regarding our health habits.

Menopause can be almost as frightening and bewildering to those around the woman experiencing it, as to the woman herself. When both partners are women, things are complicated by the possibility of going through the change together or one after the other. A male partner, although not likely to experience menopause personally (although versions have been described), can be significantly disturbed by the process. He may feel a loss of control at witnessing his partner's stormy emotions. Her decreased sex drive may make him feel inadequate or undesirable. Some men won't talk about their concerns, and the woman is left out in the cold without this knowledge.

All partners take the chance of misunderstanding the symptoms of menopause for loss of love and desire for them. This confusion is so great at times, it can destroy a relationship that otherwise should have survived and grown.

The troubled significant other may be a child or parent who interferes, usually with the best intentions, but often with a bad result. I can remember a 22-year-old daughter who came in with her mother who was on estrogen therapy. The daughter was very upset. She demanded that her mother get rid of the hormones and exclaimed to me, "Why does she need them anyway?" (I've also run into cases where a mother tells a menopausal daughter, "Don't let them give you any of those hormones, now! They give you cancer!")

Clearly it is important that those partners and family members whose support we need should be involved in the evaluation and decision process, as opposed to learning about it after the fact, often from a misinformed or uninformed perspective. Hormone replacement therapy is a tough decision, and it requires a transitional process in which family support can make a significant difference.

The intimacy between lesbian couples makes them a special case. Unlike mothers and daughters, women in lesbian relationships are likely to go through menopause together, and it may be just as tough when they don't. Some studies have shown that lesbians may engage in certain behaviors that could place their health at higher risk than heterosexual women. For example, they are less likely to get screened for breast cancer or get Pap smears.

Sometimes both partners will choose to go on replacement therapy. Sometimes one chooses to go on it, and the other doesn't. Sometimes, neither wants to take it.

The influence of family, friends, and partners is so significant in terms of the way we consume and implement information, they should be an integral part of health-care decision making.

The Gospel Truth—HUSBANDS, PARTNERS, AND FAMILY: No Woman Is an Island

• • •

1. The support of a woman's partner, family, and even coworkers as she goes through menopause and her treatment, may make the difference between successful and unsuccessful transition.

2. The information family, friends, and others can provide about you can add to the evaluation and help make it more objective.
3. Same-sex partners may encounter a challenge when they experience the change differently and want to make different choices.
4. Don't ignore complaints or problems observed by your partner.

19

MENOPAUSE AND THE MEDIA
Sorting Through the Stories

●　　●　　●

The media and the Internet have become the newest health-care providers. Unfortunately, TV, newspapers, magazines, Web sites, and other nonmedical sources of information are not necessarily supervised for accuracy of information, nor are they immune from bias. The latest and greatest inventions at the cutting edge of medicine do not always translate into the best clinical approach in everyday life. Clinical trials of new treatments and medicines may not foretell problems that will occur when ordinary people use them over longer periods of time after they are released. The first couple of years of a newly released treatment often tell a different story than expected.

Unfortunately we respond to the media as an authority. Granted, the media have done a great deal to improve public access to health information, but they must be recognized as sources of information, not conclusions. Part of the problem is that when a new research project reveals its first data, it is often picked up out of context and in small pieces. This was demonstrated clearly when Viagra was released for men, and suddenly was being used by women "unofficially" because of a supposed benefit. Baby aspirin for heart disease is another good example of taking a good thing too far. Aspirin was shown to help prevent second heart attacks. This was interpreted to mean it was good for everybody. The result: aspirin-induced gastrointestinal bleeding requiring admission to the hospital and a large, unnecessary health-care expenditure.

The media are good places to be exposed to new information and can be a source of education, but that's no substitute for proper health care. Both the media themselves and their sources can be influenced by political, social, economic, and anonymous agendas. The health-care system is not immune to bias either, so a balanced input from several sources of information will serve you best.

As we saw, the advent of birth-control pills engendered tremendous negative press. As it turns out, the lower-dose pills have proven to be *safe* for most women, with some unexpected side benefits, such as decreased anemia, decreased menstrual pain, and potentially lowered risk of ovarian and other cancers. The press also neglected the fact that all the legitimate risks associated with birth-control pills are actually higher with pregnancy!

Do the media have a gender bias? Toward women? Toward men? I think a very individual assessment is required, including the type of medium and the responsible parties involved. (Stereotyping is as bad as bias.) The slant given to information can go back farther than the media reporting it, to the original source. Researchers can be so excited about potentially positive conclusions that they may rush out incomplete information, ultimately resulting in a great deal of disappointment.

The media not only influence the health information we are exposed to, but also the economics of health. The coverage for Viagra is a good example of the power of political and information persuasion. Insurance companies rarely cover alternative treatments, natural hormones, or oral contraceptives, yet they almost universally covered Viagra or prioritized the decision to cover it. Was this accidental? Did the drug companies influence the decision? Was gender preference involved? Did the media influence the outcome? These questions certainly provide some food for thought. Perhaps it will make things clearer to consider the situation in Japan, where the government only recently lifted a ban on the Pill that had been in place for over 30 years. Viagra was approved in just six months.

Whether or not an insurer chooses to cover a procedure, medicine, or specific medical condition has a huge influence on your choice. Women's health care is a pointed example. We have just won our right to annual mammography over 50 and coverage of preventative health checkups, yet getting fertility coverage continues to be a problem. Anesthesia for childbirth has been assigned as "elective" in some cases. I suspect if men had babies, this would no longer be the case.

In the struggle of the insurers to survive economically, it is a challenge to be all things to all people. But the responsibility of insurers, especially government-sponsored plans (which become models for the rest), is to advise of best health practices even if they cannot fund them completely, rather than to equate necessity with coverage. For example, if an annual mammogram is the best option current medical knowledge can determine, but it's covered only every other year, insurers should say so plainly: "We can't afford to pay for a yearly mammogram, but we still recommend it!" Give women the option to get the more frequent treatment on their own dollars, or at a discounted rate, instead of trying to pretend that the covered treatment is adequate and more screening is unnecessary. As a patient, you, too, have a responsibility, to be willing to spend on your health as a priority: You have the most to gain and to lose.

The reality is—a penny saved is a penny earned. If you prevent disease or detect it early, it's cheaper! The cost savings of HRT unfortunately do not come immediately, and may take years to become evident. This has prevented insurers from supporting improved screening and early detection.

The breast-implant scare is a good example of the effects of the quantity and quality of media reports on women's health issues. Undoubtedly, some of the women who had silicone breast implants had complications and negative immune-system responses. Some seem to even have become very ill in response to the implants. But repeated studies have not been able to show a definitive link between implants and autoimmune health problems. Is it an across-the-board problem for all women with implants? Maybe not. Some people's bodies just don't seem to accept foreign materials as well, which could be a clue to the discrepancy in complications. Organ transplants are another example: Some patients' bodies do not reject transplants as readily; others quickly reject the donor organ, despite powerful anti-rejection medications.

After the media covered all the lawsuits, settlements, and frightening complications, women rushed to their plastic surgeons to have their implants removed. It was almost like a "run on the bank." But most women's concerns were unwarranted. If a woman who has had silicone breast implants has had no particular health problems since, I would not recommend removing her implants. It is worth neither the risk of another surgical procedure nor the cost.

HERS and PEPI Studies

The media publicizes medical research daily. The initial results of the HERS (Heart and Estrogen/progestin Replacement Study) and PEPI (Postmenopausal Estrogen/Progestin Interventions) studies were released recently to much media fanfare and much misinterpretation by the press, the public, and some caregivers as well.

HERS was a clinical trial to evaluate the effects of hormone replacement therapy on women who had already had a coronary disease "event." (Event: a nice way to say "heart attack.") It was intended to determine the effectiveness of estrogen and progestin in preventing a second event. Contrary to expectations, the hormones did not seem to reduce the risks of either death or a nonfatal heart attack in the first four years of use. (In fact, there seemed to be an increase in such events during the first year, but a slight decrease by the fourth and fifth years.) These results were very surprising to many, and were widely misinterpreted by the public to mean that estrogen increased the risk of heart attacks for all women. But there are two important reasons that that conclusion cannot be drawn. First, the women in the study all had heart problems. Perhaps estrogen is better at preventing the onset of heart disease than at protecting those who already have it. Second, the study was a relatively short one; it's possible that the benefits, which began to show up after four years, are for the long term. Additional research, as always, is needed to determine the real meaning of the early study results, and to follow these women for a much longer time.

The PEPI trial studied symptom relief and the side effects of hormone replacement therapy in healthy, postmenopausal women. It found that hormone therapy significantly reduces hot flashes and heart disease while increasing bone density, and that including some form of progesterone in the therapy assists in uterine health. Despite this good news, the PEPI results seemed to receive much less media attention than the HERS study. This shows that one important aspect of media fairness is consistent access to information. It is not enough to report objectively on any one study; we need the ability to weigh multiple studies as they are released. The mostly favorable recommendations of PEPI were reported by some of the media, but without the hue and cry that greeted the HERS studies, despite the broader range of the former.

On the Horizon: Other Studies

The MORE (Multiple Outcomes of Raloxifene Evaluation), RUTH (Raloxifene Use for the Heart), WHI (Women's Health Initiative), and WISDOM (Women's International Study of Long Duration Oestrogen after Menopause—oestrogen is an alternate spelling of estrogen) studies are all due to release results sometime after the year 2004. All are intended to provide further evidence of the usefulness of selective estrogen receptor modulators (SERMs) in treating menopause and its related symptoms. MORE will study raloxifene in general, while RUTH will study raloxifene and its potential cardiovascular benefits. The WHI and WISDOM studies will both examine estrogen and hormone replacement therapy in general.

Help! My Insurance Won't Pay for My Treatment!

As the health-care situation in this country deteriorates, it is becoming harder for women to get quality care in general and for menopause and its symptoms in particular. Proper treatment requires *time* with a professional, and that is becoming a scarce commodity. There are a few areas where more comprehensive media coverage might help make the public aware enough (or outraged enough) that some positive change may actually occur:

- Medicare just stopped paying for certain laboratory tests they consider unnecessary. For example, they currently will only pay for one Pap smear every three years. Most insurance companies don't cover the newer, more accurate Pap smears available (such as PapSure).
- Not too long ago, pain relief for labor was considered elective by some insurers. Can you imagine their not paying for pain relief for a vasectomy?
- Insurance coverage of medications, particularly natural compounding, varies. A lot of the newer therapies may not be covered. Most insurance plans covered Viagra almost immediately, but birth control and hormones are still not widely covered.
- Most of the time, diagnosis and treatment are billable under normal insurance, but compounding and other specialized treatment may not be. HMOs rarely have the resources or time to spend on these treatments.
- Most medical insurers don't pay for osteoporosis screening, or will only pay for one evaluation in a lifetime, despite the fact that a comparison bone scan is the only way to know if treatment is working. The insurers think they are saving money, but in the long term, the cost of osteoporosis disability and treatment will be exorbitantly high. The medical insurers figure you'll be covered by Medicare by the time you get screened, so it won't be their problem. Medicare inherits the higher costs of the late complications and reduces the coverage or access.

The Gospel Truth—MENOPAUSE AND THE MEDIA: Sorting Through the Stories

• • •

1. Because the news media often reports on the latest study findings and medical reports without any in-depth analysis or knowledge of the context and mean-

ing of the reports, each story should be treated as incomplete information, not as a recommendation.

2. The medical community needs to take a stronger leadership role in presenting good information to the lay public.

3. Medical treatments for "female problems" are treated as more elective than those for men.

4. The medical insurance and HMO industries, as well as the media, also exhibit gender bias, whether admitted or not.

5. Because of rising costs and political agendas, some coverage, such as osteoporosis screening and Pap smears, face reduced payments from many insurers, including Medicare. Some new tests won't be covered at all.

20

HOW ESTROGEN PLAYS WITH OUR BODIES
Other Pieces of the Puzzle

• • •

Estrogen has an influence on almost every organ system in the body. Most of us are aware that estrogen influences the breast, the uterus, and other reproductive organs. But before you began this book, did you know estrogen affects the proper functioning of the brain and neurological system, the skin, the bones and joints, sexual functioning, the heart and blood-clotting system, the colon, the endocrine system, the liver, and the gallbladder?

In the proper amounts and at the right time, estrogen generally maintains the proper function of these systems, and facilitates their interaction with other organ systems. On the other hand, with harmful sources, incorrect dosages, inappropriate timing, or in an at-risk or pre-sensitized individual, it may cause skin pigmentation, fluid retention, blood clots, liver disease, gallbladder disease, uterine and breast cancers, and blood-sugar irregularities.

For example, birth-control pills—which may contain estrogen in ten times the potency of estrogen replacement therapy—can pose significant risks, particularly in women who smoke. Alternatively, low-dose replacement therapy, which does not provide birth-control benefits, is not responsible for the same degree of complications, and in some cases doesn't carry these risks at all. Women who have trouble with nausea on birth-control pills won't necessarily be nauseated on hormone replacement therapy. Headaches, especially migraines, may be aggravated by oral contraceptives and improved by estrogen therapy.

Your age, the type of estrogen, source of estrogen, dosage, duration of treatment, and regimen all significantly affect results, side effects, and complications. Tailoring to the individual woman is the name of the game.

Let's discuss some more specific effects of low estrogen levels on body systems. (Some of the following body systems have already been covered in their own chapters, so are only mentioned here in summary.)

Brain: As discussed previously, low estrogen may cause loss of memory, irritability, depression, lack of concentration, and fogginess. There is a reduction in the incidence of Alzheimer's disease with women when on replacement therapy, which points to even more complex, far-reaching effects.

Skin, hair, and nails: A multitude of reported effects, such as: wrinkling and dryness of skin; hair and nail breakage; lack of vaginal lubrication; painful sexual intercourse; hair loss; facial hair growth; and loss of sense of smell. Many women dread more than anything the onset of coarse facial hair. As with men, it seems that hairs lost from the head spring up in unwanted places. It appears notably on the chin and upper lip, but can occur on any part of the body that you least desire it. They are often bristly hairs that are hard to remove. (Try waxing or electrolysis.) Many women are also surprised when their pubic hair falls out during perimenopause; it's disconcerting, but normal. Sometimes it grows back, sometimes not.

More severe hair growth or loss needs an endocrinological workup, regardless of age.

Hormone replacement therapy influences hair growth in these ways:

- Estrogen affects the rate of growth and the start of new growth. Hair may become finer and lighter in tint.
- Progesterone compounds have no real, direct effect although increase in fuzzy facial hair has been reported.
- Androgens (male hormones) increase the coarseness of each hair, except on our heads. (Too bad—they aren't a cure for baldness.) They also contribute to facial hair growth.

Your skin also has estrogen receptors. During perimenopause and after menopause, your skin will undergo changes in texture and thickness as its estrogen supply dwindles. It may become thinner and dried out. Estrogen returns plumpness to the skin and may smooth its texture, restoring a more healthy appearance. Wrinkling appears to increase in the absence of estrogen.

Collagen is a vital substance in your body that keeps your skin and tissues supple, elastic and full. As you age, your body loses collagen at the rate of 2.1 percent per year, starting usually somewhere in your early 40s. Eventually, your skin becomes dryer and less pliant. Estrogen helps to reduce the rate of collagen loss.

Eyes: After the age of 40, the eyes' lenses may begin to lose elasticity. Hormone deficiency may have a relationship with certain disturbances of vision and may cause dry eyes as well. All the mucous membranes become drier. Glaucoma may be unrelated to hormones, but the incidence increases above age 40, so women should have their eyes checked every three years starting at age 40, every two years if they have a family history of glaucoma or already wear glasses, and every year if they are severely nearsighted. There is some evidence that macular degeneration, a serious eye condition, may be decreased by estrogen use.

Heart: Symptoms of low estrogen include flushing, palpitations, chest pressure, rapid heartbeat, and arrhythmia.

Urinary tract: Problems with irritable bladder, urgency, and bladder infections are common. Loss of urine with coughing (incontinence) may become worse.

Endocrine system: There are effects on blood sugar, calcium, metabolism, and other parts of this system.

Skeletal system: Osteopenia, osteoporosis, decreased flexibility and nonspecific aches and pains in bones and joints are common complaints.

The breasts: Lack of hormones can cause breast tenderness. Some women experience an increase in breast pain.

Uterus: The uterine lining is the tissue that develops and is shed during your monthly period. Estrogen builds it; progesterone sheds it. Low estrogen levels can cause the uterus to dry up and fail to maintain healthy tissue. However, where the uterus is concerned, low estrogen levels are not as problematic as high estrogen levels. Estrogen can increase the growth of fibroids, which are benign muscle growths in the uterus and occasionally in the ovaries. It can cause pain, and may cause the lining to become too thick if not used in conjunction with progesterone. Estrogen can promote the growth of endometriosis or reactivate it. This is a condition when the lining of the uterus travels through the fallopian tubes and implants inside the abdomen outside the uterus, often causing bleeding and scar tissue. Ovaries are common sites to find implants.

Mythical Effects

• • •

Estrogen is commonly blamed for some effects it does not have:

- It has not been proven to increase the risk of ovarian cancer.
- It does not increase the risk of uterine cancer, when administered with progesterone.
- It does not cause fibrocystic disease of the breast.
- It can be the cause of migraine, but it can also be the cure.
- It can be the cause of breast pain, but it can also be the cure.
- It can also be both the cause and treatment of abnormal bleeding.
- It does not cause blood clots with the same incidence as birth-control pills.
- It does not cause significant weight gain in the proper doses.

Ultrasound imaging can measure the lining through new, refined techniques, which helps to determine the body's estrogen level, and screen for precancerous change of the organs. If the lining is too thick (greater than 5mm), then a biopsy may need to be done in the office to rule out problems. Sonograms or ultrasound are painless and very informative. Progesterone is responsible for shedding this lining naturally as a period when we're younger, and artificially when taken cyclically (10–13 days a month) when we are on replacement therapy. Progesterone can also prevent a lining from developing at all if taken continuously (daily).

As long as estrogen is balanced with progesterone, or the uterus is absent, the risk of cancerous change can be largely eliminated. It's important to remember that this risk may be present whether the estrogen is synthetic, natural, over-the-counter, chemotherapeutic, or by prescription. Monitoring is necessary regardless of the source of estrogen. And of course you can still get uterine cancer without taking hormones.

The following chart describes the effect on the various organ systems of having too much or too little estrogen.

Organ System	Too Little Estrogen	Too Much Estrogen
Cardiovascular	palpitations, fatigue	fatigue, increased blood pressure, swelling
Reproductive	infertility, vaginal dryness, loss of orgasm, irregular bleeding, uterine cramping, uterine bleeding	abnormal bleeding, abdominal swelling, increased secretions, ovarian pain
Neurological	loss of memory, irritability, migraine, nervousness, depression	irritability, restlessness, insomnia
Skin, hair, and nails	dryness, easy damage, hair breakage, nail thinning and breaking, skin "crawlies"	excess moisture and vaginal discharge, flushing, swelling, weight gain, bloating
Musculoskeletal	muscle fatigue, leg cramps	swelling, muscle aches
Breasts	breast tenderness, decreased breast size	breast tenderness, breast enlargement, breast swelling, itchiness of nipples

The Gospel Truth—HOW ESTROGEN PLAYS WITH OUR BODIES: Other Pieces of the Puzzle

• • •

1. Estrogen affects almost every organ system in the body, including the brain, skin, hair, nails, eyes, heart, digestive and urinary tracts, endocrine system, reproductive system, skeletal system, and the breasts.

2. Generally, estrogen can have a positive effect on all the organ systems it affects, but with incorrect dosages, inappropriate timing, harmful sources, or in an at-risk or pre-sensitized individual, it may cause more health problems than it helps.

3. It has not been proven to increase the risk of uterine cancer or fibrocystic breast disease or to cause weight gain when taken properly.

4. By balancing estrogen with progesterone, the risk of cancerous change to the uterus can be eliminated.

5. Estrogen can both cause and cure migraines, abnormal bleeding and breast pain, depending upon the source, the sensitivity of the individual, and the dosage of estrogen.

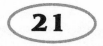

FORMS AND METHODS
A Guide to Dosage Adjustment and Forms of Administration

• • •

If you are experiencing side effects, adjusting the dosage or changing estrogen type can solve most problems. The "art" of dosage adjustment comes from your doctor understanding the nature of your problem and being familiar enough with your physical makeup and the options available to help you make the change smoothly. Here are some common side effects and possible solutions:

Problem   **Then Try . . .**

Weight gain   Lower dosage, different brand, fitness and nutritional evaluation with food diary, exercise.

Retaining water   Decrease dosage.
Skipping one to two days a week of estrogen.
Increasing vegetables and fruit.
A mild diuretic to help flush some water from your body.

Nausea   Try with full stomach.
Change time of day of dose.
Switch type of oral agent.
Try a non-oral agent, such as the patch.

Bleeding   Evaluation of lining of the uterus with ultrasound and endometrial biopsy to rule out fibroids, polyps, precancerous change, or uneven thickening of the uterine lining. (Must be done first if not done recently.)
Decrease or increase dose.

Problem	Then Try . . .
	Changing progesterone/estrogen balance. Other sources of bleeding, such as the bladder and vaginal area need to be checked. The bleeding pattern is an important clue, such as mid-cycle versus continuous bleeding early or late in the cycle, as well as the cyclic or continuous regimen variations.
Breast pain	If breast pain occurs after starting therapy, it may subside spontaneously within two to four weeks, so wait it out. If the pain becomes worse after starting therapy, an adjustment in either progesterone or estrogen needs to be accomplished, most likely by lowering dosage. (Progesterone is the more likely culprit.) Vitamin E—approximately 800 IU to 1000 IU—may be helpful; it's not proven, but it is also not harmful. Restricting caffeine may help, too. If there is an associated lump, or a current mammography is not available, a mammography should be performed. Pain is usually not a sign of cancer but should be ruled out. Breast ultrasound may also be helpful if cystic breast disease is present.
Vaginal dryness	Sometimes the vaginal area does not receive the same estrogen as other areas of the body through oral or transdermal routes, either due to dose or distribution. The solution is to add a small amount of estrogen cream locally to improve moisture immediately and facilitate comfortable intercourse. Consideration can then be given to raising the oral dose to overcome the lack of moisture in the vaginal tissue if no other side effects are created, especially if continued use of cream is inconvenient. Estring, the vaginal ring, is another option for treatment.
Hot flashes	Estrogen levels can be assessed to determine if you are absorbing your dosage or clearing it too rapidly. If so, adjusting to a non-oral route with follow-up monitoring to determine adequacy of absorption or too-rapid clearance may be successful. Problems with blood sugar, thyroid, and other conditions should be tested for, to eliminate other possible causes of similar symptoms. Sometimes, splitting the dose is necessary (taking half the dose twice a day, instead of a single daily dose), because hot flashes may be more frequent during a certain time of day.

Problem	**Then Try . . .**
	Although the dose should last 24 hours, it does not always. Sometimes progesterone and testosterone can be added to decrease the symptoms.
Headaches	Too much or too little estrogen or progesterone can cause headaches, but more often, headaches are caused by acute relative changes in levels of either hormone. Environmental triggers, such as certain foods, or stress can cause them. If they are hormone-related they can usually be dealt with by decreasing or increasing the dose, and changing from oral regimens to transdermal systems, or from continuous instead of cyclic regimens.
Aches and pains in bones and joints	Some individuals are sensitive to natural animal substances in a particular estrogen, or its binding agent or colorings, which may cause an allergic phenomenon; therefore, switching brands of estrogen may solve this problem. (The red dye in Premarin, for example, has been a source of allergy.) The sensitivity or allergy may manifest as pain in the joints, rashes, and/or stomach upset. Conversely, if aches and pains were present before therapy, they may have been caused by other mechanisms, and may be resolved by therapy.
Losing hair	Hormone changes can cause hair to get thicker, become very thin, or to break more easily, depending on the degree of the change. Try increasing your estrogen, or lowering your testosterone.
Nervousness and agitation	Usually a sign of intolerance to estrogen, which can sometimes be handled by dose adjustment, or changing the source of estrogen.
A persistent rash under the transdermal estrogen patch	This is usually a reaction to the adhesive used to attach the patch to your skin. If the patch is satisfactory in all other ways, try to "fan" the patch after you peel it open, before applying, allowing the alcohol (which may be an irritant) to evaporate. This may not help as much with matrix-type patches. You can also put a small amount of over-the-counter cortisone cream on the irritated area, after removing the patch. You may be able to reduce the rash or prevent it by rotating the patch site. Never place the patch in the same location twice. The ring around the patch is very difficult to remove. Use an adhesive remover to avoid rubbing the skin too hard. A change in brand may work, because the adhesive or other components may vary somewhat from patch to patch.

Problem	Then Try . . .
	As a last resort, you may have to switch to another method if the rash persists.
	A compounded gel or cream may have the same beneficial bypass of the gastrointestinal tract without the allergic side effects, as does sublingual (under the tongue) dosing of certain types.
Patch seems to wear off before time to change it	Sometimes your patch may need to be changed more frequently than recommended, and/or you may have to wear a larger-dose patch, or wear two patches to get the right level of hormones.

If at any time you change your diet, which may change your nutritional level of estrogen, you should inform your doctor so it can be taken into consideration. Ditto for over-the-counter supplements. Taking vitamins can either increase or decrease the hormones' effects.

Forms of Administration

Estrogens come in oral tablets, sublingual tablets, skin patches, injections, or compounded creams and gels. There are almost as many varieties as cosmetics. These include:

- Oral tablets—Taken by mouth and swallowed.
- Sublingual—Placed under the tongue and allowed to dissolve.
- Transdermal patch—Attached to the skin and absorbed.
- Gels—Applied locally and rubbed in.
- Skin creams—Applied locally and rubbed in.
- Suppositories—Inserted into the vagina and allowed to dissolve.
- Vaginal creams—Inserted into the vagina via an applicator with a plunger.
- Injections—Injected directly into the body.
- Subdermal pellets—Inserted under the skin and absorbed slowly over time.
- Vaginal ring—Inserted into the vagina and left to release medication slowly.

Nonsystemic or local therapies are those that have little or no effect on the rest of the body, including vaginal tablets, vaginal creams, and the estrogen ring (Estring). (If you use a large dose of estrogen vaginally, however, you will have a systemic (bodywide) effect.) These therapies are often chosen when you are unwilling to accept even a low risk of more estrogen, or need especially quick local relief. For example, vaginal cream relieves dryness and makes intercourse more comfortable in the first few uses.

There are two basic regimen styles:

Cyclic—This regimen involves taking estrogen part of the month, and estrogen plus progesterone part of the month, sometimes with a break without either hormone. This allows the build-up of the uterine lining and then shedding, somewhere toward the end of the estrogen/progesterone combination, or on the break if there is one. The number of days of progesterone will typically range from 10 to 13. The days will be arbitrarily assigned for convenience, for example, from the first to the tenth of the month, resulting in a period mid-month. If periods are still regular, we can assign the days to coincide with the existing natural cycle. Bleeding will occur at the end of the progesterone/estrogen cycle, or up to five to seven days later. Any day after the twentieth day of the cycle, bleeding can occur and is considered normal.

Here are some examples of common cyclic regimens:

Estrogen Days	Progesterone Days
1–30	21–30
1–25	16–25
1–25	13–25
Monday–Friday	1–10

Continuous—A continuous regimen involves taking your dose of estrogen and progesterone on a daily basis. This prevents development of the uterine lining and periods altogether, although "breakthrough bleeding" can occasionally be a problem for up to six months. A variation is taking estrogen and progesterone Monday through Friday, with a weekend break from the hormones for people who are sensitive and cannot tolerate a sustained dosage. This can help reduce breast tenderness or bloating but may cause breakthrough bleeding or symptoms over the weekend.

Patients who are younger and perimenopausal, and still having period activity, typically use cyclic regimens. The continuous regimens, although they can be used at any time, are most effective after periods are light or have ceased. Whether you choose cyclic or continuous you can take hormones in any form: pills, patches, creams, etc. A woman who still has her period but wants to try the continuous method must be prepared to endure irregular bleeding for up to six months.

Both methods—cyclic and continuous—are safe. Both methods require evaluation of abnormal bleeding.

Some women can't tolerate a full dose of progesterone or any at all. These women need an aggressive supervision plan, including ultrasound measurement of the uterine lining and biopsies of the lining. This will help prevent precancerous and cancerous changes from unopposed estrogen. A measurement of 5mm or less from an ultrasound reading is considered very unlikely to be cancerous. Any abnormal bleeding warrants an office sampling or biopsy.

Bypassing the Liver

Women who have liver damage or liver disease may need hormone replacement methods that bypass the liver, such as transdermal (through-the-skin) patches or creams, rather than pills. Patches may also be preferable for someone who takes tranquilizers or other drugs, or drinks heavily . . . anyone with too much stress on the liver.

The Gospel Truth—FORMS AND METHODS: A Guide to Dosage Adjustment and Forms of Administration

● ● ●

1. Hormone replacement therapy can be as much an art as a science. It is critical to adjust the balance of the hormones being administered, and to follow up

during treatment so side effects can be minimized and desired effects can be optimized.

2. Some methods of dosage adjustment include: lowering the individual dose, "cycling" the dose (skipping days); trying a different brand or formulation; switching the type of dose (such as from oral to patch); splitting the dose; taking the dose at a different time of day; or, changing the balance of the hormones being taken. All compromises have benefits and risks.

3. Changing your diet may increase the nutritional sources of estrogen and should be taken into consideration. Similarly, taking vitamins may influence some hormone side effects and can increase or decrease the hormones' effects.

4. Women with liver disease or liver damage should consider transdermal hormone replacement therapies, which bypass the liver.

5. All abnormal bleeding needs evaluation.

22

KEEPING IT ALL TOGETHER
When, Where, How Often, and Why

• • •

Many times, women come to me with difficult questions. So often in life, people tell us these types of questions have "no easy answers." In my practice, I'm truly fortunate in that there are easy answers—many of them. The problem is, just because the answers are easy, that doesn't make them easy to follow through on! For example, one of the easiest answers I can give women who ask me how to improve their quality of life, reduce their risk of cancers, reduce their risk of heart disease and stroke, and make their menopause years much easier is to give up smoking. Easy to say, but not so easy to do. If at first you don't suceed, try, try again. There are no demerits for how many times it takes.

With that truth in mind, here is my easy guide to keeping it all together, health-wise:

• Get an annual checkup.
  An annual examination should be viewed as a wellness and prevention opportunity. Many of the illnesses that women experience are preventable and if caught early, treatable. You should have Pap smear and blood pressure checks every year, and mammogram and blood-stool checks once a year after 40. Blood evaluation of cholesterol, triglycerides, kidney function, electrolytes, blood count, thyroid, and blood-sugar evaluation should be taken every other year after 40. Have a

bone-density evaluation between age 50 and 65 (depending on risk factors), with follow-up as indicated. Don't forget eye exams and hearing tests.

- Don't smoke.

  If you don't smoke, don't start. If you do, quit. If you can't quit, cut back. Smoking is the only factor other than genetics that is proven to affect the age of menopause. Smokers, even former smokers, can reach menopause two or more years earlier than nonsmokers.[27] The number of diseases, causes of death, etc., you expose yourself to when you smoke is endless. Use the patch, the gum, the pills, or just go cold turkey. Stop feeling guilty—just quit!

- Don't drink.

  Although it's fine to have an occasional glass of wine, the idea that you can drink regularly without any ill effect is not true. You may have heard that a glass of wine is good for the heart, but this benefit is probably outweighed by the risks of: increased breast cancer, injuries while under the influence, increasing complications of pregnancy, and fostering addictive potential for those who have a genetic predisposition to it.

- Don't do drugs.

  As with smoking, if you don't take them, don't start. If you use them, quit. This includes traditional, nontraditional, and over-the-counter drug abuse.

- Exercise.

  Try to get some form of regular exercise for at least 20 minutes, three times a week, and work up to 30 to 40 minutes, three to five times a week. Find something fun that you can look forward to, rather than dreading it. Keep it simple if your life is busy. Walking works wonders. Avoid high-impact activities for prolonged periods of time, such as jogging, or anything that jars your bones and joints, because over a long period of time it causes arthritis and other chronic injuries. Focus on low-impact and relaxing activities; yoga is a fabulous way to stretch, relax, and remain limber throughout your later years.

- Take care of your teeth.

  Visit your dentist as least once a year. Floss and brush regularly. As you age, the quality of your life stays higher when you have your own teeth. Estrogen helps prevent tooth loss.

- Take care of your eyes.

  Get an eye exam every two to three years, and always wear UV-protected sunglasses to guard against harmful ultraviolet light. The incidence of cataracts is diminished with adequate eye protection. If you are diabetic, or if you take steroids, make sure you are checked annually.

- Wear sunscreen.

  With our diminished ozone layer, and our sun-worshiping lifestyle, the incidence of skin cancer is on the rise. Wear a lotion with an SPF (sun protection factor) of 25 or better every day, particularly on your hands, face, and other exposed areas. Even incidental exposure on your arms and face when you are driving is significant. Sun exposure without protection accelerates wrinkling as well.

- Protect your hearing.

  Many of you have already bombarded your ears with loud concerts in your youth, and didn't know you could permanently damage your hearing. Avoid loud noises and persistently loud music. The better you protect your hearing, the more likely you won't need a hearing aid at a young age or at all. If you do need a hearing aid, don't resist it. You'll miss hearing a lot.

- Take a bubble bath once a week.

  It does wonders for your ability to rejuvenate, reduce stress, and renew your lease on life. Light some candles and have a glass of sparkling mineral water with a twist of lime.

- Get rid of toxic relationships.

  If you're with a partner or have a parent or child who is abusive to you, whether it be physically, mentally, or spiritually, get out of the relationship. You deserve to be happy. No one deserves to be treated badly, *no matter what.*

- Wear a seat belt.

  One of the most senseless causes of death and disability is

being in an automobile accident without a seat belt. Even if
you exercise and your diet is low-fat, your windshield doesn't
know the difference: If you're not buckling up, you're wast-
ing your time.

- Practice safe sex.

  Just because you feel safe, it doesn't mean you are safe. It
  doesn't matter how old you are, how young you are, how
  well you know each other, if it's "only once," or how negative
  your blood tests are, the risk is still there, and it's not worth
  dying for.

- Don't drown in guilt.

  Guilt is a wasted emotion that has been built into our psyches
  through centuries of socialization, and serves no purpose. It
  may be impossible to rid your life of guilt entirely, but try not
  to be dominated by it.

- Follow a reasonable diet.

  Try to stick to a low-fat—but not no-fat—low-salt diet with
  plenty of fresh fruits and vegetables. Keep it balanced and
  avoid extreme regimens and radical weight-loss plans. Take a
  reasonable amount of vitamin and mineral supplements.
  Extreme megadoses may be flushed out of the body and
  down the toilet, and they may do you harm. More is not always better.

- Listen to music.

  (But not too loudly . . . see "Protect your hearing," p. 183.)
  Expose yourself to a variety of music, dance, and art in different settings. Cultural pursuits regenerate your spirit and
  stimulate creativity. You will be a more interesting person.

- Do everything in moderation.

  Excess in any area of your life limits your success, but that is
  not to say you shouldn't take risks and pursue your dreams.
  Don't spend your senior years saying, "If only I had . . ."

- Spend time with your partner and family.

  As Ferris Bueller said, "Life goes by pretty fast and if you don't
  stop once in a while and take a look around, you could miss
  it." Hug, hold hands, and touch each other as much as possible. When the opportunity passes, it may not return again.

- Laugh.

  Laugh as much as you can, at yourself and with others . . . not at others. Use your stress to make positive changes rather than negative. There's no such thing as getting rid of stress, but laughing helps you cope with it.

- Read.

  Books, magazines, fiction, nonfiction, poetry. Read it all. If the eyes are the windows to the soul, reading is the window to the outside world. It keeps your mind sharp, active, and open.

- Manage your negative emotions.

  If you're angry, get help to work through it, because it will eat you alive. If you're sad and hopeless, get help! There are many reasons it happens, and lots of ways to restore you to your normal life and good feelings. Don't waste any more time.

- Say no.

  Learn to say no when you can't do something, or don't want to do something. You'll resent people less by being honest with yourself and them.

- Manage your time.

  Leave a little earlier than you think you need to, and try to arrive places ahead of schedule. Rushing to get somewhere when you're late is a major cause of unnecessary stress and accidents. Be realistic about time expectations.

- Have faith.

  Whether it be traditional religion or not, nurture your spiritual needs. Have faith in yourself, because no one should believe in you more than you do. If you believe in yourself, the world will treat you as you desire and expect.

The Gospel Truth—Keeping It All Together: When, Where, How Often, and Why

• • •

1. Be good to yourself.
2. Be safe.

3. Moderation!
4. Forgive yourself.
5. Think happy. Be happy.
6. Time is short.
7. If at first you don't succeed, try, try again. There are no demerits for how many times it takes.

23

CHOOSING YOUR HEALTH CARE TEAM
When Bad Doctors Happen to Good People

● ● ●

Frances, a 35-year-old television editor, tells of an experience she had when, at the age of 18, she decided to get her first gynecology checkup. She was getting serious with her boyfriend, and they were planning to get married soon. She thought it would be a convenient time to discuss birth control, to make sure that she was healthy, and to begin a relationship with her physician for the future. Needless to say, she had the usual anxiety that most women have about this interaction, and delayed it as much as possible.

As Frances remembers it, everything went wrong.

"I didn't have insurance, and they told me, 'You better bring the money in when you come, because we don't work for free around here.'

"When I got to my appointment, the waiting room was drab and dreary, with worn-out furniture and ancient, tattered magazines. The room was filled with women waiting to be seen. I had to fill out a stack of papers an inch thick. I don't know why they couldn't have sent them to me before my appointment.

"Finally, they took me to the exam room, where they gave me a tiny paper gown and made me wait even more. The exam itself was rushed, cold, and impersonal, and the doctor didn't even give me a chance to ask any questions.

"I got dressed, slowly. I was sort of in shock. I went to the front desk,

having had none of my questions answered, having had no educational materials offered to me about my concerns, and having an overall feeling of having been completely ignored. No, worse than ignored; I felt as though I had been violated.

"And then, before I left, I had to write out a check for $250."

Frances's story is all too typical. Unfortunately for too many women, it is the rule rather than the exception.

I founded our woman's health-care center in Southern California in 1985 to improve what is often described as one of the worst experiences a woman goes through. I did this by creating a women's health center where the facility is warm and appealing in both its environment and its staff, and where the first priority was quality health care delivered in a nurturing environment.

So, what is reasonable for you to expect?

It's okay to expect to be seen in a reasonable amount of time. It's okay to speak up when you're being made to wait. It's okay to take control of the situation. You shouldn't be afraid, intimidated, or too frustrated to call the office or to talk to the office personnel when you're there.

The success of a health-care experience is affected by the environment and by the relationships between the patient and the physicians and staff almost as much as the care itself. An effective wellness and prevention program depends on a true partnership between patient and doctor. When you are undergoing treatment, this is even more true.

The physician you select is a critical factor in making the decision to pursue estrogen therapy. It goes without saying that your provider should possess the appropriate training and degrees, and have a reputation as someone who won't overintervene or undertreat. If you have any questions about a physician's credentials, just ask.

This individual needs to be well-read, open-minded, a good communicator, and relatively accessible. Your physician's team of front-office assistants, nurses, covering physicians, and support personnel need to be of high caliber, motivated to care for you with caring and kindness, as an individual.

You, too, have great responsibility in making this relationship more effective and successful in maintaining your health and detecting disease. You must be honest and straightforward in providing your history. You must be prepared with written questions so they may be answered, and to remove any doubt you may have, because this could affect the success of your therapy. If you have decided not to take a particular replacement or medication, be straightforward about that choice.

You have the responsibility of keeping your physician's office staff apprised of current addresses and phone numbers, so they may reach you with test results, or in an emergency. It is frustrating and dangerous when something abnormal happens.

The doctor has a responsibility to inform you properly of test results, particularly abnormal ones. For example, calling on a Friday afternoon and leaving a message on your answering machine is a no-no! You will spend all weekend worrying about it, unable to see the doctor or consult with a surgeon or specialist.

You need to encourage participation by providing information about your therapy to your significant others. If they have questions or concerns, your physician should be aware of them, especially if they may affect your willingness to continue with therapy. A joint visit can sometimes alleviate miscommunications that may otherwise interfere with successful treatment. Often the more you can keep your partner involved with your physician's decisions and your treatment plan, the more likely he or she is to be supportive of whatever decisions you make. Your partner and your coworkers are also an important part of monitoring the progress of your treatment plan.

You have the task of following instructions and, if you deviate from the plan, of clearly notifying your physician; otherwise, he or she will have no way of knowing what is working or not working in your treatment. It is also important for you to follow health-care screening guidelines at appropriate intervals. In other words, while you may be under a doctor's care for menopausal symptoms or a breast lump, you still have the same risks of developing other conditions. Continue to have the recommended screening tests.

The physician and his or her staff have a responsibility to make you comfortable in the office setting. It goes without saying that physicians must be well educated, with training specific to women's health, but they also have to be able to talk with you on a level you can understand.

You must be treated courteously, on the phone and in person, and you should accept nothing less.

The front office must be flexible in offering appointments and scheduling enough time for your expected needs. They shouldn't treat you as if you're required to address them by military rank or salute. No generalissimos or sergeants need apply!

The office should be clean, decorated with warmth and caring. Reasonably recent magazines and reading material should be available in the waiting room to ease the tension while waiting, which should be kept to a minimum whenever possible. If your mother recognizes the magazines from her first visit years ago, there may be a problem . . . If your mother's still waiting from her first visit, there's definitely a problem!

At no time should you fear rescheduling or frequent calls to the office when they are needed. The staff is there to serve your needs.

Physicians and allied health-care providers should be on time as much as possible and if late, the delay should be communicated to the patient with alternative options offered. The patient's privacy and confidentiality should be protected at all costs. Matters personal to you should never be revealed in a loud voice, in public areas, or to inappropriate people. You should never have even the slightest concern for your safety.

The office should have appropriate attire for your examination, including adequate size and length of examination room gowns, and reasonable temperature of surroundings. The décor of rest rooms, examination rooms, and so on, should not be reminiscent of a laboratory environment.

The physician and staff should make eye contact at least some of the time while you're talking to them. You should not be made to feel embarrassed, guilty, foolish, or inappropriate at any time. There is no such thing as a stupid question. You should feel open to share your feelings and concerns. It's also really nice when people remember you and address you by name.

Finally, barring a life-and-death concern, you should be

supported in your decision making even if it disagrees with your physician. You should always feel free to get a second opinion on any issue of concern, and a good physician never minds another colleague's opinion.

All of these factors toward creating a strong physician-patient relationship are important with any health treatment, but they may be especially important with hormone replacement therapy, because it is long-term therapy. To reap all of the available benefits, you must remain on estrogen for several years; three is considered a bare minimum in most cases. Some women take it for the rest of their lives. It is important to have a physician who will look after you during these years, and who will keep up with the ever-increasing range of options for your treatment.

Frances now comes to our practice. She is a little older and whole lot wiser. "Now, I go to a practice that is much more in tune with my needs," she says.

"Even the small things make all the difference in the world, because no screening test or health prevention works if you are too afraid to go to your physician to receive it. Fortunately for my daughter, her experience will be a much better one and will create a more positive basis for her ongoing health care throughout her lifetime."

The Gospel Truth—Choosing Your Health Care Team

• • •

1. Most women have negative experiences for their first gynecological exam that may prevent them from returning for years.
2. Many women continue to have negative experiences when they get their annual exams.
3. Women have the right to expect to be treated well when they visit their doctors, and should demand respect, timeliness, explanations of treatment, and courtesy.
4. Physicians have a responsibility to ensure the com-

fort, safety and good treatment of their patients. It is the physician's duty to be sure the patient leaves the office feeling informed and well treated.

5. The office should be clean and comfortable.

6. Office staff should be professional, courteous, and respectful of patients' privacy and the potential for discomfort.

24

NOW, IT'S UP TO YOU
Recommendations and Decisions

● ● ●

"To take estrogen or not to take, that is the question. Whether to suffer the slings and arrows of osteoporosis and heart disease or to get dreaded breast cancer?"

—Ms. William Shakespeare?

So, you've almost finished this book. You've read the stories. You've related to the symptoms. You're anxiously looking forward to checking out the appendices, checking the wellness screening charts, and taking the Hormonal Balance Quiz. You've perhaps said to yourself as you've read along, "That's exactly what I'm going through!" Or, maybe you just like to read the end of a book first, and that's okay too.

What now?

What do you do now that you're up to your eyebrows with information about your body, your health? What if, like the women in some of these stories, you've tried everything already and it hasn't worked? What if your doctor's office is like the one described in Chapter 23? Or, on the other hand, what if your doctor is really good, and has been helpful and supportive in the past, but, you fear, just doesn't have enough information, resources, or facilities to help in your particular case? What do you do?

1. Find the right provider. Word of mouth is invaluable to help you find a good doctor—ask your friends in the same age

group, especially those friends who seem to be content with their medical care and whose opinions you respect. If you cannot find an appropriate doctor through word of mouth, contact the North American Menopause Society (*see Appendix F*), or your local hospital's referral services and ask for a referral.

2. Start keeping the diary or symptom journal in Appendix C for a month before your checkup. This will document clearly where you are starting from.

3. Make a list of current health problems and the medications you're taking and bring a copy to your checkup. Don't forget any over-the-counter products and supplements you are taking; these can be more important than your regular medications.

4. Make a list of all hormones and birth-control pills you've taken in the past and the side effects or complications you've had with them. Note the dates of starting and stopping them.

5. Bring all the info to your selected provider. If you feel a mesh of your personalities, and his or her advice seems reasonable, begin following it.

6. Insist on being monitored at least every 2–3 months until you've found complete balance, free of side effects. After that, return for at least a once-yearly assessment; sooner if there is a change in symptoms or health.

7. Follow the health recommendations in Chapter 22, "Keeping It All Together."

8. On the back of your journal pages, keep track of the visits, side effects, change of medications, and any new health problems. Your life is busy—don't rely on memory. You will learn a great deal about yourself with the exercise.

If you have a primary-care physician or HMO you are happy with, but feel you are not getting anywhere regarding your hormone therapy or menopause treatment only, you may choose to see a specialist for a short time to get on the right track. When your problems are settled, you can return to your primary-care physician to continue follow-up and implementation.

The Estrogen Decision—How to Make It

There have been many facts and figures in this book that I hope will aid each individual woman in making the best decision for her circumstance. It won't be easy, and it may not be right the first time. An understanding of how we arrive at decisions regarding health care and what influences those decisions is essential to getting the best results.

As we have stated many times, heritage and its culture exerts a profound influence. There may be certain biases that have been reinforced that augment our interpretation of what's good for us. These messages are introduced from the time we are born to the present, from family relationships, the media, and community input. If your second grade teacher said you couldn't sing or your mother said your ears are too big, you never forget it. It's likely you never sing in public and your hairstyle always covers your ears. Even when scientific fact may disagree with the style or substance of our cultural leanings, those leanings still influence us. Sometimes, rather than abandoning the past in favor of current or future ideas, a blending of these worlds works best. Even the health statistics of a particular group of people or a region are profoundly influenced by their immediate environment and cannot be transposed to a new place with the assumption that nothing will change. These influences include nutrition, style of living, degree of stress, genetic predisposition, and exposures to toxins or pollutants. Our genetic makeup is the canvas on which we paint our individual paintings.

We are always limited somewhat by what we started to work with. Genetic engineering may change our canvas at some future time, but for now the genetic makeup our bodies are born with forms a basic starting point we cannot escape.

Experience then molds the genetic base with cultural overlays and environmental influence into a blended individual. What we survive, encounter, or endure profoundly changes our behavior. As we've previously discussed, a negative early interaction with physicians, hospitals, medications, or illnesses forever changes our perceptions. A striking example of this is the woman whose mother had, or even worse, died of, breast cancer. Her approach to health issues will always be overridden with this grave and appropriate concern. Her risk is somewhat higher, but she also associates habits and choices her mother made with her death, whether reasonable or not.

Such a daughter may react by getting regular checkups, self-examining her breasts monthly, religiously getting her mammograms done, and reading all she can about the disease. Alternatively, the same experience may cause another daughter to shun medical attention, skip self-exams, and have mammography reluctantly, if ever. Her fear will prevent health-protective behaviors and interventions, even at the risk of her own life, due to her family's negative personal experience.

So what do we do? Objectivity, particularly in hormone decision making, is important. The approach requires us to analyze any past influences and bring them to the forefront of our awareness. Sneak up and shake your fears. Dealing with those feelings and their resulting biases is the first step toward a stronger, comfortable decision framework to work from. Sometimes it will also take great patience and the passing of time.

Education is also very important. Reading materials, videos, media presentations, and other sources of good learning material are invaluable to balancing bias with fact. Even biased materials are okay as long as you expose yourself to both sides. The more information in your arsenal, the better, even if it is occasionally confusing.

Self-study in whatever form, such as keeping a journal of your present perceptions and subsequent actions on a daily basis, will help tremendously in identifying the best approach for you to follow personally. Part of this process should include a personal pro-and-con list to be added to with the help of your health-care professional: What's good and what's bad about hormones for us as individuals and in the eyes of professionals we trust. This journey of self-realization makes it easier for all involved to reach the best choice at that time. The decision will be influenced by personalized family risk factors, personal viewpoints, availability of treatment options, and the level of trust you have with the physician or other health-care provider.

After you have created your list and a journal of your symptoms, begin assessing your options. Try to form as complete a list as possible of the hormone replacement options as well as alternative, non-hormonal options with your feelings, positive or negative alongside. Leave room for regular updates.

Example:

Choice	Pros	Cons	Feelings
Oral estrogen	Osteoporosis protection. Cardiovascular disease protection. Stop hot flashes.	Possible increase in bleeding. Taking a pill.	*(Enter your feelings, positive or negative, and why.)*
(Enter your other options here.)			

At the completion of this analysis, along with expert professional guidance, most women will reach comfortable conclusions on how to proceed. It is a working plan that should be dynamic and flexible as your needs change, rather than a rigid schedule.

Whether you choose estrogen or not, this will help you stay objective. You can change your mind when circumstances change. It's your life, and it is always your decision, pro and con. Do the homework and the outcome will be worthwhile.

Absolute Contraindications to the Use of Estrogen

It is important to note there are cases or conditions where a woman may not be able to consider estrogen at all, or should wait until the condition is rectified before proceeding. These include:

- Recurring or active thrombophlebitis (inflammation of certain blood vessels, accompanied by pain and swelling) or thromboembolisms (lung clots and leg clots)
- Suspected breast cancer
- Undiagnosed uterine bleeding
- Active liver disease

Additional reasons women may feel uncomfortable taking estrogen, or their physicians may not want to prescribe it, that should be considered but are not strict contraindications include:

- Certain other liver problems
- Gallbladder disease
- Endometriosis
- Uterine fibroids
- Migraines
- Personal or family history of breast cancer
- High triglycerides

What Makes Women Quit Estrogen

If you have tried estrogen before and quit the program, you are not alone. The things that cause most women to quit estrogen are fairly consistent over a wide sampling. Knowing these in advance can help you to deal with them better, and work with your doctor to eliminate or prevent them. They include:

- Fear of cancer
- Abnormal uterine bleeding
- Breast pain

- Breast cancer
- No history or symptoms of bone loss or heart disease
- Too much time between physician appointments (not enough reinforcement)
- Complicated replacement regimens
- Inconvenience
- Expense
- Weight gain
- Headaches or dizziness
- Changes in the shape of the eye (Sometimes these changes make it difficult to wear contacts, or the contacts need to be refitted as a result.)
- Other side effects
- Social issues (i.e., fear of dependency on a drug, tendency to view menopause as a tradition, not a disease, peer pressure)

Gallbladder disease, certain liver or kidney conditions, and asthma are things that many people think are contraindications to estrogen use, but they are not necessarily so.

Lupus, a connective tissue autoimmune disease, also benefits from estrogen.

Women are much more likely to stick with their treatment plans if they understand the potential for reduced risk of broken bones, heart disease, Alzheimer's, and the possibility of improved mental functioning.

We also find that women are more likely to stick with estrogen if they experience the following while on therapy. Again, advance awareness can help you to work with your physician to increase the likelihood of these things happening:

- A diagnosis of osteoporosis, confirmed by bone-density testing
- Close monitoring
- Individualized dosage regimens
- Alternative routes (forms) of administration available
- Open attitude toward natural products
- Regimens that eliminate periods, not bring them back

As you think about the ideas and practices discussed in this book, try to identify the areas of greatest concern to you and ask your doctor how to work around them. For example, if you are particularly concerned with weight gain, you might discuss how to optimize your exercise or diet simultaneously with beginning any hormone therapy and take your weight out of the equation. Although we cannot prepare for everything that may happen in the course of therapy, if we attempt to look after what we can, it may give us more latitude if something unexpected happens.

THE FUTURE
A Vision

●　　●　　●

Stop and imagine what you would like to see in the future regarding health care. The possibilities are overwhelming! Let me tell you what I imagine. I would like to see more research into how to reduce our biggest health risks, and how to make our interventions and therapies safer and more effective. (The old adage that the cure is worse than the disease is still true in some cases.)

I think we would all agree that improvements in screening techniques are needed. I've often wondered what went on in the minds of the inventors of the mammogram. Did they have pieces of fruit to squash as models? Would they have designed this method to test for testicular cancer? (All kidding aside, it happens to be the best we've got right now, and should be utilized according to the guidelines to increase your chance of early diagnosis and cure.) New on the horizon are tests that are based on Magnetic Resonance Imaging (MRI), refined ultrasound, and new markers that will light up abnormal cells so they can be imaged clearly even when they are very small.

Even better, through refined genetic testing and genetic engineering, one day we will augment our defenses before disease even starts. And when we better understand the interrelationship of genetics and environment, our ability to prevent rather than treat disease will be greatly enhanced.

The Pap smear, which is only 50 to 60 percent effective in picking up abnormal cells, is being improved as I type. PapSure, a new visual test, picks up abnormal cervical cells at a rate of an additional 30 percent or more. This makes screening 90 percent effective or better. Rather than collecting cells from a woman's body for observing in a lab, the PapSure test allows your health-care provider to perform an internal examination of the cervix and vaginal canal "live." Detection of abnormal cells is immediate, and is more precise than traditional Pap smears. Another new test, called Thin Prep, is similar to a traditional Pap smear, but is also more reliable.

In the future we will be able to identify precancerous viruses and inactivate or kill them before cell damage occurs.

Certainly, we all look forward to the day that sigmoidoscopy and colonoscopy (intestinal exams where an instrument is inserted into the rectum to look for colon and other gastrointestinal cancers) are replaced.

Sexually transmitted diseases may one day be prevented by vaccines or oral agents or both. These new treatments could kill offensive organisms on contact, preventing infection completely.

Perhaps someday our delicate hormone balance will be measured when we are born, during adolescence, and in our childbearing years, using tests that will set the parameters for hormone replacement in the future. We will then also learn to manipulate our natural hormones if our genetics put us at risk. For example, what if our natural estrogen levels have been too high since our adolescence, placing us at an increased risk for breast cancer? We might choose to change the level of estrogen early enough to stop the changes. Although we already classify certain types of women at high risk, we don't really know what types or levels of hormone are safe for them, or when and what is really dangerous.

As both home and workplace become more democratic in outlook, stress will be greatly reduced. Respect and appreciation will cross the barriers of gender, culture, and age. Worthwhile endeavors for work and satisfying work environments will become more and more commonplace. Those of us who choose to dedicate periods of time to raising our children will garner as much recognition as working women for our contributions to our society and our families. Women will have no fear of sexual assault or violence in the home. We will become better drivers, always wearing seat belts and driving safer cars.

Our increasing awareness of the importance of education will help abuse of alcohol and drugs to become nonexistent, as we prepare our children and families to remove the need for these dangerous substances. Genetically, we will determine who is at risk and avoid exposure in the people most vulnerable.

New hormones that continue our progress—better defining the receptor functions and improving the efficacy and side effects—from raloxifene, tamoxifen, and the other "designer estrogens" will be introduced. These drugs will be even more selective, stimulating only the organ receptors desired and none of the receptors that are not. We could individualize each regimen, giving women a risk-free therapy that will free us to enjoy our postmenopausal years without fear, without loss of health, and with exuberance for the future.

Advances in infertility, prenatal, and postnatal care are bringing nearer the day when the decision to have a baby will be available to all women who choose it. Pregnancies will be better monitored and the outcome for both Mom's and baby's health will be enhanced. Perhaps it's not too far a stretch of the imagination to dream of the end of labor pains, episiotomies, and tears during delivery.

Better medications that help headaches, especially migraines, but don't cause dangerous or intolerable side effects will be widely available. Improved low-risk alternatives to hysterectomy (which will be performed only on women who need them) will be introduced and readily available. Better options for treating breast cancer—and, better yet, sophisticated prevention—are on the distant horizon. Superior tests to watch our bones and effective treatments that prevent them from dissolving before we're done with them will surely be available well before the end of this century. We will have the ability to keep our minds sharp and our emotions positive, so we may enjoy all these advances in our lives.

The elderly and very ill can look forward to better care, with improved pain medications and access to support services.

And while we're at it, let's not forget the elimination of high blood pressure, diabetes, and heart disease. If we're lucky, we'll see cigarettes become extinct, instead of us.

In this rose-colored future, the design of workouts, nutrition, and supplements would be individual, easy to maintain, and allow you always to reach your personal goals. Our society will revel in our diversity on all levels. I do not wish for a "brave new world" of identical perfection in all of our lives. I would like, however, our human variety to be exemplified by our interests, our colors, our shapes, our art, our music, our writing—not the array of diseases and suffering we can get and already have.

If and when this vision will become real, how, and in what order, no one can tell. I think we can all join together to share the dream of better health care, and a better world for our children and grandchildren for generations to come.

THE DRUGS THEMSELVES
Dosages, Brand Names and Types

●   ●   ●

There are several different "forms" or methods for taking the various hormones that have been discussed in this book. They are potentially natural, synthetic, animal, or plant. Some of these treatments may be used in an "off-label" fashion; that is to say, they may be used in a way other than was originally intended by the manufacturer. For example, a hormone that was designed to be swallowed as a tablet may be used sublingually (under the tongue); or the dosage may be modified to provide more effective results.

Types of Estrogen

Estrogen forms may be single or blended with progesterone or testosterone, continuous or cyclic.

- Tablets or capsules (oral)
- Transdermal (patches)
- Creams (vaginal or skin)
- Vaginal ring (vaginal)
- Subdermal implants (under-skin pellets that dissolve over time)

Types of Progesterone

Progesterone forms may be cyclic or continuous, in various intervals from five times a week to once every three months.

- Tablets (usually oral)
- Capsules (oral)
- Gel (skin)
- Cream (skin)
- Lotion (skin)
- Injection
- Suppository (rectal or vaginal)
- Rectal suspension enema

Types of Testosterone

Testosterone may be taken every day, three times a week, or less.

- Lozenge (dissolved in mouth next to cheek)
- Capsule (oral)
- Sublingual tablet (under the tongue)
- Gel (skin)
- Cream or ointment (skin)
- Injection

BRAND NAMES, DOSES, AND FORMS

Here is a list of some of the brand names and forms for the different hormones and other important treatments:

Oral Forms

Estinyl—Ethinyl estradiol. 0.02, 0.05, 0.5mg. A synthetic source of estrogen, Estinyl is considered somewhat "old-fashioned," but works for some women.

Estrace—0.5mg, 1.0mg, 2.0mg. Great for breast tenderness. It was originally intended to be swallowed, but it works very well sublingually as an "off-label" use.

Estratab—0.3mg & 0.625mg tablets (synthesized from soy and yam plant sources).

Estratest—Esterified estrogens and methyltestosterone tablets, 0.625mg estrogen/1.25mg testosterone; 1.25mg estrogen/2.5mg testosterone. Good option for increasing libido and other testosterone-deficiency symptoms. The testosterone does not convert to estrogen.

Evista—Raloxifene HCl, 60mg tablets, taken daily. This SERM (selective estrogen receptor modulator) is a good choice for women with few overt symptoms who want bone and heart protection.

Metronidazole is not a hormone, but a commonly prescribed treatment for various types of vaginal infections. It can be given as oral tablets, brand name Flagyl, or as a local gel, brand name Metrogel.

Ogen—Piperazine estrone sulfate. 0.3, 0.625, 1.25, 2.5, 5mg.

Orthoest—Piperazine estrone sulfate. 0.3, 0.625, 1.25, 2.5, 5mg.

Premarin—Estrogen, in 0.3, 0.625, 0.9, 1.25mg Premarin tablets; Premarin Vaginal Cream; Prempro conjugated estrogens/medroxyprogesterone acetate tablets, 0.625mg/2.5mg and 0.625mg/5mg; Premphase conjugated estrogens/medroxyprogesterone acetate tablets, 0.625mg/5mg (cyclic). Premarin is the most studied and prevalent estrogen. Many report conclusions are extrapolated from studies of Premarin to other sources.

Promensil—Estrogen, obtained from red clover. 40mg tablet. All four estrogenic isoflavones.

Prometrium—Progesterone, USP 100mg capsules. Prometrium is an oral, micronized progesterone. When replacement therapy is given continuously, we use 100mg daily; in a cyclic regimen the dosage is 200mg. It is the first natural progesterone available orally that can survive the acid in the stomach. If you are sensitive to progesterone, this may be an alternative. Some women are more sensitive to natural than synthetic, so don't be surprised if your side effects are in fact worse. Some women can't tolerate progesterone in any form. As with most new medications, insurance may not pay for this source of progesterone yet.

Transdermal Estrogen (Patches)

Alora—Estradiol transdermal patch. 0.025, 0.0375, 0.05, 0.1mg. Changed twice a week.

Climara—Estrogen, estradiol transdermal system. 0.05mg/day, 0.075mg/day, 0.1mg/day. Climara is a good choice for those who are sensitive to estrogen in high levels, and/or who like to change patches only once a week.

CombiPatch—Estrogen, estradiol/northindrone acetate transdermal system. Estrogen plus progestin transfusing the skin. CombiPatch eliminates the need for oral progestin. Can be used cyclically by alternating with a nonprogestin patch.

Estraderm—Estradiol transdermal patch. 0.025, 0.0375, 0.05, 0.1mg. Vivelle is now considered a better form of patch.

Fempatch—Estradiol transdermal patch. 0.025, 0.0375, 0.05, 0.1mg. The Fempatch offers a wide variety of dosages with an alternative adhesive. Changed twice a week.

Vivelle—Estrogen, estradiol transdermal system. 0.375mg/day, 0.05mg/day, 0.075mg/day, 0.1mg/day. Better than Estraderm. This form has an improved adhesive and "matrix" style of delivery.

Other Forms

Estring—Vaginal ring. 2mg/(7.5mcg/daily). Works for 90 days. Especially good for delivering very-low-dose estrogen to women with vaginal symptoms. Estring is appealing because it is not messy and lasts longer than creams. A choice to consider for breast cancer survivors.

Compounded Formulas

Oral triestrogen and biestrogen are usually available in 1.25, 2.5, 3.75, 5.0, and 7.5mg capsules.

You can figure out the equivalent dose by multiplying the traditional dose by four.

For example, a traditional dose of 0.625mg of Premarin equals 2.5mg of triestrogen or biestrogen (0.625 x 4 = 2.5).

Estriol alone is available as a cream at 0.5 percent, and as a pill in 2, 5, 10 or 15mg sizes.

Testosterone

The following forms of testosterone are all useful in treating loss of libido and energy associated with androgen deficiency.

Testosterone Proprionate—Vaginal ointment, applied to the skin ¼ tsp. once or twice a day.

Natural Testosterone Lozenge—Orange- or mint-flavored lozenges; 5mg lozenges, taken as half a lozenge (2.5mg) dissolved between the cheek and gum three to five days a week.

Testosterone Gel—Applicator (syringe). 0.5 to 1.0ml applied daily to the skin of the thigh or abdomen. Use on the upper arm should be avoided, to keep the gel away from the breasts.

Testosterone gel is a 4mg/ml (0.4%) solution and is used in doses of 0.5 to 5ml daily, massaged into the wrist, thigh or abdomen. Dosage changes should not be done any more frequently than two to three weeks. Maximum increase will be 1.0ml daily.

Testosterone ointments, gels, or creams are 1 to 3 percent solutions, and are blended in a semiliquid compound, used externally. This treatment is usually used directly on the vulva area once or twice a day. The dose is usually ¼ teaspoon. The amount also can be decreased over time when benefits are realized. Some clitoral enlargement may occur, and should be reported for a decreased dosage adjustment or change of therapy. Avoid contamination of the urethra area and vagina because the ointment is not soluble.

Progesterone

Progesterone can be taken in a cyclical regimen with estrogen, as described earlier, or separately, in the following forms:

Micronized Oral Capsules—In an oil base. 25mg, 50mg, 100mg.
Sublingual Oral Capsules—In an oil base. 25mg, 50mg, 100mg, 200mg.

Sustained-release tablets without oil.

Vaginal Suppositories—25mg, 50mg, 100mg, 200mg, 400mg, 800mg.

Progest—Cream. 1.5% (over-the-counter), 5%, 10% (prescription). The low dosage is recommended for women with mild symptoms; the higher doses are for women with more noticeable symptoms.

Other Transdermal Creams—1%, 1.5%, 3%, 5%, 10%.

COMMONLY PRESCRIBED ANTIDEPRESSANTS

Selective Seratonin Reuptake Inhibitors (SSRIs)

Celexa (Citalopram)

For: adult patients with depression or severe depression
Disadvantages, Side Effects: vomiting
Drug Interactions: Metopolol, Macrolides, Azole antifungals
Dosage: 20–40mg/day
Availability: 20mg, 40mg tablets

Luvox (Fluvoxamine)

For: obsessive-compulsive disorder (OCD)
Disadvantages, Side Effects: use limited to OCD, nausea, sexual dysfunction
Drug Interactions: Warfarin, Hismanal, Seldane, Carbamazapine, Bezodiazepines, Halperidol, erythromycin, Quinidine, Verapamil
Dosage: 50mg HS
Availability: 50mg, 100mg tablets

Paxil (Paroxetine)

For: adult patients with major depression, panic disorder, obsessive-compulsive disorder (OCD)

Disadvantages, Side Effects: constipation, dry mouth, sexual dysfunction

Drug Interactions: Cimetidine, penytoin, tricyclic antidepressants

Dosage: 20mg/day for depression, 40mg/day for panic disorder and OCD

Availability: 10mg, 20mg, 30mg, 40mg scored tablets; 20mg, 30mg film-coated tablets

Prozac (Fluoxetine)

For: adult patients with major depression, bulimia nervosa, obsessive-compulsive disorder (OCD)

Disadvantages, Side Effects: insomnia, agitation

Drug Interactions: Buspar, tricyclic antidepressants

Dosage: 20mg/day for depression, OCD; 60mg/day for bulimia nervosa

Availability: 20mg/5ml liquid; 10mg, 20mg capsules

Zoloft (Sertraline)

For: adult patients with major depression, panic disorder, OCD

Disadvantages, Side Effects: maintenance dose is 2–4 times initial dose, diarrhea

Drug Interactions: Warfarin, tricyclic antidepressants

Dosage: 50mg/day for depression, OCD; 25mg/day panic disorder

Availability: 25mg, 50mg, 100mg scored tablets; 25mg, 50mg, 100mg capsules

OTHER ANTIDEPRESSANTS

Wellbutrin (Bupropion)

For: adult patients with major depression, patients unable to tolerate SSRI antidepressants

Disadvantages, Side Effects: high incidence of seizures with rapid release form, headache, nausea, agitation, insomnia, dry mouth, constipation

Drug Interactions, Contraindications: history of seizure disorder, bulimia or anorexia nervosa

Dosage: 100mg twice a day or 75mg three times a day

Availability: 5mg, 100mg film-coated tablets

Remeron (Mirtazapine)

For: adult patients with major depression

Disadvantages, Side Effects: somnolence (drowsiness), dry mouth, weight gain, increased cholesterol and triglyceride levels

Drug Interactions, Contraindications: Diazepam, history of agranulocytosis

Dosage: 15mg/day

Availability: 15mg, 30mg capsules

Serzone (Nefazodone)

For: adult patients with major depression associated with anxiety

Disadvantages, Side Effects: sedation, P450 inhibition

Drug Interactions: Seldane, Hismanal

Dosage: 100mg twice a day

Availability: 100mg, 150mg, 200mg, 250mg capsules

Effexor (Venlafaxine)

For: adult patients with major depression

Disadvantages, Side Effects: sexual dysfunction, gastrointestinal upset, cardiovascular side effect

Drug Interactions: MAO inhibitors, Cimetidine

Dosage: 75mg/day in 2–3 doses

Availability: 25mg, 37.5mg, 50mg, 75mg, 100mg capsules

APPENDIX B

HERBAL AND NATURAL PRODUCTS
Common Names, Dosages, and Indications for Use

•　　•　　•

The natural, botanical, and herbal products listed here are commonly used for treatment of symptoms of menopause.

Name (Source)	Claimed Benefit	Comments or Recommendation
Black Cohosh (herbal)	Reduces hot flashes, eases PMS and cramps	May interfere with estrogen, since it may contain phytoestrogens.
DHEA (natural)	Reverses effects of aging	Needs study. Many claims are unproven and overblown. Side effects are not known, but has been linked to liver cancer.
Dong Quai (herbal)	Relieves cramps.	Many negative side effects and contraindications. Not recommended.
Echinacea (herbal)	Boosts immune system, anti-inflammatory, antiviral	Taken in tea infusions, tinctures, fresh or dried, or in pill form. Contraindicated in chronic progressive diseases such as tuberculosis and AIDS.
Evening Primrose Oil (herbal)	Breast tenderness, PMS, hot flashes	3 grams a day. Be aware that products usually contain vitamin E as well. Your total dose of vitamin E should not exceeed 1000mg/day.

Name (Source)	Claimed Benefit	Comments or Recommendation
Feverfew (herbal)	Controls migraine headaches	Taken as dried leaves (25mg) or powder (82mg to 1–2g). Can accentuate anticoagulant activity. May interact with some medications.
Fish Oils (natural)	Natural estrogen (potential benefits of estrogen)	2–3 servings a week.
Flaxseed (botanical)	Plant estrogen (potential benefits of estrogen) and omega-3 fatty acids	1 to 3 tablespoons in dry form, or a few teaspoons in oil form.
Garlic (botanical)	Reduced cholesterol and serum lipids and reduced blood pressure	Claims not substantiated. Few adverse effects—rarely causes nausea, sweating and light-headedness. May interact with anticoagulants.
Ginger (botanical)	Antinausea, antivomiting. May lower pain of rheumatoid arthritis	Avoid during pregnancy. 940mg of powdered ginger 25 minutes prior to motion sickness exposure may reduce symptoms.
Ginkgo Biloba (herbal)	Mental sharpness, improves circulation, decreases anxiety and depression	Commonly used for memory loss, supposedly increases blood flow to the brain. May increase bleeding time or clotting time.
Kava-Kava	Mood elevator.	May cause a skin rash.
Soy (botanical)	Plant estrogen (potential benefits of estrogen)	One serving (40mg) a day.
St. John's Wort (herbal)	Mood elevator (antidepressant)	Should not be mixed with prescription antidepressants. May irritate stomach; take with meals, per directions. May cause photosensitivity.

If you take anticoagulants, aspirin, or ibuprofen, avoid taking any of the following botanicals: alfalfa, cinchona bark, clove oil, gingko biloba, garlic, ginger, ginseng, and feverfew.

If you are taking antidepressants, avoid ginseng, ma huang, and St. John's wort.

VITAMINS

Note: You'll see a wide variation in dosages for some of the following vitamins, minerals, and other nutrients. The correct dosage for you depends largely on your health, diet, lifestyle, and the needs of your body. Consult with your own doctor to help determine what is best for you.

Vitamin A

Benefits: Deficiency of vitamin A can cause blindness. Excess may cause gastrointestinal upset and liver disease. It is absorbed better with fat in food. Vitamin A may help boost the immune system and help fight breast cancer, and may help insulin effectiveness. Vitamin A derivatives are in Retin A, the acne and antiwrinkle cream.

It is difficult to overdose on vitamin A via diet, but it is possible with supplements. Sources of vitamin A include carrots, cantaloupes, and leafy greens.

Dose: The recommended daily allowance of Vitamin A is 3,300–4,000 IU/day. It can be toxic in large doses: More than 5,000 IU/day is not recommended. Beta-carotene, which converts to vitamin A in the body, may be taken up to 10,000 IU daily.

Vitamin B1 (Thiamin)

Benefits: Aids in carbohydrate metabolism and neurological function. Sources of B1 include brown rice, dried beans and legumes (including soy), egg yolks, and wheat germ.

Dose: 1–50mg/day.

Vitamin B2 (Riboflavin)

Benefits: Vitamin B2 helps with red blood cell formation and antibody formation. It is found in meat and dairy products, beans, spinach, and cruciferous vegetables, such as broccoli and Brussels sprouts.

Dose: 1.2–50mg/day.

Vitamin B3 (Niacin, Niacinimide)

Benefits: Aids conversion of fats and protein into glucose.

Dose: 100mg/day.

Vitamins B5 (Pantothenic Acid) and B6 (Pyridoxine)

Benefits: Although all the B vitamins are helpful, B5 and B6 in particular are thought to minimize water retention, ease various symptoms, and reduce effects of stress. Estrogen may increase the need for vitamin B6 in the body. Sores around the mouth are a sign of B6 deficiency. Vitamin B6 may help relieve morning sickness, and may help reduce heart disease, strokes, and depression.

Dose: B5, 100mg/day. B6 1.5–100mg/day. It should be noted that high doses of B6 (more than 100mg/day) are associated with risk of nerve damage.

Vitamin B12 (Cobalamin)

Benefits: Vitamin B12 deficiency is associated with depression, nerve symptoms, and pernicious anemia. A substance called "intrinsic factor" is necessary for you to be able to absorb vitamin B12.

Dose: 2.4–400mcg/day. B12 is especially important for vegetarians. It should be used with folic acid for maximum benefit. If your body doesn't make enough intrinsic factor, you may need shots or nasal spray to be able to absorb the vitamin.

Vitamin C

Benefits: Vitamin C may lead to lower risk for cancer and heart disease, and has been linked to reduced risk of stroke. Serious vitamin C deficiency has been linked to an increased risk for disease, including scurvy, a degenerative disease of the gums and skin. Vitamin C is an antioxidant.

The benefits of vitamin C are increased when it is taken with bioflavinoids, such as Hesperidin.

Dose: 200–500mg/day. It can be found in many foods, especially citrus fruits, as well as supplements. It is water-soluble, and will pass through the body if taken in large doses. It is not advisable to take more than 500mg/day without supervision, as overdoses can cause diarrhea, gas, and bloating. It is becoming more common for people to take large doses of vitamin C, but the benefits are still being studied.

Vitamin D

Benefits: Vitamin D can help bone strength, and is needed to enhance the absorption of calcium. Sunlight exposure is necessary to naturally maintain vitamin D levels.

Dose: The recommended daily allowance is 200–400 IU, which can be achieved with 15 minutes of sun a day or a supplement. Vitamin D intake of as much as 600–800 IU is recommended to reduce risk of fracture in older women, especially if they do not get regular exposure to sunlight. Vitamin D may be toxic in large doses, so avoid taking more than 1,000 IU per day.

Vitamin E

Benefits: Vitamin E may help hot flashes and breast tenderness and may be beneficial for preventing coronary artery disease. Vitamin E is an antioxidant.

Dose: 400–1,200 IU of vitamin E daily has been used to control hot flashes. It should be noted that some studies have found no benefit, but it also acts as an antioxidant, so is still useful in those doses.

At high doses, vitamin E has some negative effects on blood-clotting activity, as well as other toxicity, which should be avoided. It may have some negative effects on bone mineral density as well. Do not combine vitamin E with aspirin or gingko biloba at high doses, because of an increased risk of bleeding troubles.

Vitamin E comes in gel capsules, tablets, and oil.

Vitamin K

Benefits: Aids in reducing blood clotting.
Dose: 25–60mg/day.

TRACE ELEMENTS

Boron

Benefit: Boron helps metabolize magnesium. It may have some effect on your hormone levels. There are some claims that it may help with hot flashes. Boron works best in combinations with magnesium, manganese, and calcium.
Dose: 1–3mg/day.

Other useful trace elements include fluoride (3.1–3.8mcg/day), manganese (2–5mg/day), molybdenum (150–500mcg/day), silicon (5–10mg/day), and vanadium (10mcg/day).

MINERALS AND NUTRIENTS

Calcium

Benefit: Calcium is critical for bone strength. It helps maintain bones and teeth, aids nerve transmission, may lower blood pressure, and helps heartburn.
Dose: Menopausal women who are not taking estrogen should

take 1,800mg–2,000mg of calcium a day, while women taking estrogen should take 1,000–1,500mg/day. More than 2000mg/day is not recommended, because it may interfere with absorption of other minerals. Calcium doses should be achieved in combination with dietary sources, by eating foods rich in calcium. Typically, supplements with calcium carbonate have the highest elemental calcium, but some people have stomach distress (such as gas and burping) with calcium carbonate. Try other forms such as lactate, citrate, or gluconate if you have trouble with calcium carbonate. These other forms are absorbed differently by the body, so be aware of the total elemental calcium you are receiving.

Your body absorbs calcium better when it is taken with food. Splitting the dose by taking half the dose twice a day, or one-third the dose with each meal, improves your body's ability to absorb the calcium and reduces the potential for gastric upset. If you are over 65, calcium citrate is better for you because of the lower stomach acid and poorer absorption associated with aging.

Chromium

Benefits: Chromium may enhance weight loss. It is often included in over-the-counter, "natural" diet pills. Chromium can help maintain blood-sugar levels and decrease lipids.

Dose: 25–200mcg/day. 200mcg/twice a day if you have weight loss or sugar problems. May cause gastrointestinal upset; take with food.

Folic Acid

Benefits: Folic acid is an essential chemical that provides several apparent benefits to the body. It may reduce the risk of cardiovascular disease, colon cancer, and birth defects.

Dose: The recommended dose of folic acid is 400–800mcg/day, which can be easily reached with a multivitamin supplement that contains it. Folic acid should be taken with vitamin B12. Dosage may be increased to 1g/day during pregnancy. It may be taken with or without food.

Lecithin

Benefits: This substance acts as an emulsifier for vitamin E. It is an essential substance in the body, naturally occurring in the cell membranes. It protects against cardiovascular disease.

Dose: 200–500mg/day.

Magnesium

Benefits: Magnesium is a factor in bone strength.

Dose: 500–750mg/day.

APPENDIX C

YOUR JOURNAL
A Self-Evaluation Screening Chart

● ● ●

Daily charting increases your awareness of physical and emotional signs and symptoms that may help you and your health-care provider diagnose and follow treatment. Using the following chart, record and observe patterns using the suggested monitors. Add any other symptoms you're experiencing in the blank spaces and score them also. Use the journal to record periods, dietary intake, and any other potential triggers.

It is important to log your symptoms every day if possible, at the same time of day. Score the symptoms by severity from 0 to 3, 0 being none and 3 being most severe.

If you can, begin your journal one month before you go to your checkup, and continue keeping it as your therapy begins. Use the back of the journal to keep notes on your appointments, medications or change of medications, doses, side effects, and any new health problems. As we have said throughout the book, using a journal is a key factor in identifying the severity of your hormone disturbances as well as other patterns that need attention.

Scoring of Symptoms: 0 = None   1 = Mild   2 = Moderate   3 = Severe

Month: ....

DATE	1	2	3	4	5	6	7	8	9	10	11	12	13	14	15	16	17	18	19	20	21	22	23	24	25	26	27	28	29	30/31
HOT FLASHES																														
SWEATS																														
SLEEP DISTURBANCES																														
BLEEDING CHANGES																														
HEADACHES																														
TENDER BREASTS																														
DRYNESS																														
ACHES/PAINS																														
DECREASED SEX DESIRE																														
TIRED–LOW ENERGY																														
FREQUENT URINATION																														
HEART PALPITATIONS																														
HAIR CHANGES																														
MOOD SWINGS																														
TEARFUL																														
NERVOUS																														
IRRITABLE																														
ANXIOUS																														
DEPRESSED																														
UNABLE TO CONCENTRATE																														
DIFFICULTY MAKING DECISIONS																														
MEMORY TROUBLES																														
LEG CRAMPS																														

APPENDIX D

VITAL STATISTICS
How to Measure Your Success

• • •

There are so many numbers involved in health care. Your blood pressure, cholesterol, hormone levels . . . it can get overwhelming or confusing to keep track of them all! Following are some of the more important numbers you may want to keep track of. Don't rely on memory; after (or during) each visit to the doctor, write down all the numbers in a notepad or chart. By doing so, you will have a more understandable record of your health status and more concrete information you can use toward tailoring your health care to your needs.

FSH (follicle stimulating hormone) Testing: An FSH reading of greater than 20–25 IU/mL is considered high and indicates you are probably menopausal. A reading greater than 55 is considered very high, and a reading of 80–100 IU/mL is extremely high.

Thyroid: A normal TSH (thyroid stimulating hormone) reading is considered between 1 and 5 IU/L. The level of TSH goes up when thyroid is low.

Estradiol: A level of 60–100pg/mL is considered therapeutic when you're on replacement therapy (meaning it's normally balanced with what you're taking). Depending on other factors, ranges of treatment may be from 40 to 250pg/mL. This is because not all women's symptoms are controlled in the therapeutic range.

Recommended medical testing intervals for adults:

Type of Test	How Often
Blood Pressure	At least once every 2 years.
Cholesterol	Every 5 years after age 20. Every 2 years at age 40.
Fecal Occult Blood Testing	Yearly after 50. (May be done at various intervals between 40 and 50 depending on risk.)
Hearing	Routinely at doctor's discretion, or if you show symptoms of hearing loss.
Mammography	Every 1 to 2 years after 40, annually after 50.
Rectal Exam	Every 2 years between 40 and 50. Every year after age 50.
Sigmoidoscopy	Every 3 to 5 years beginning at 50.
Vision	Once every 3 years, every 2 years if wearing glasses or family history of glaucoma, every year if severely nearsighted.

Optimal lipids levels for adults:

Lipid	Optimum Level
Cholesterol	Less than 200mg/dl
HDL	Greater than 50mg/dl
LDL	Less than 130mg/dl
Triglycerides	Less than 200mg/dl
Cholesterol/HDL ratio	Less than 3.7

APPENDIX E

CHECKING YOURSELF
Your Personal Hormonal Balance Quiz

● ● ●

Answer the following questions about yourself:

- Are your periods becoming more irregular, either too close together or too far apart, lighter or heavier?
- Are your skin, hair, and nails becoming drier, changing in texture, breaking more easily, or decreasing in amount?
- Have you lost interest in sex?
- Have you noticed vaginal dryness, and/or have you had more frequent infections, vaginal tearing, or painful sex?
- Do you have trouble sleeping?
- Have you started having headaches, or, if you've had them before, have they become worse?
- Are you depressed, moody, or irritable or if you have always been somewhat depressed or moody, has it become worse lately?
- Have you started having worsening PMS (premenstrual syndrome) symptoms, or is your PMS lasting longer and starting earlier?
- Have you ever had night sweats (waking up in the middle of the night, perspiring profusely), or hot flashes (a feeling of warmth inappropriate to the environment)?
- Do you lose urine when you laugh, cough, sneeze, or exercise?
- Do you have a "hump" in your upper back (dowager's hump)?

- Have you broken a bone too easily?
- Have you noticed an increase in aches and pains in your bones and joints?
- Are you having problems with your memory that you've been chalking up to old age? (So-called senior moments even though you are less than 70 years old.)
- Has it been more than a year since you've had a menstrual period?

If you answered "no" to all of these questions, you probably have not started perimenopause yet.

If you answered "yes" to one to three questions, you may just possibly be beginning the perimenopause. Consider consulting with your doctor to determine your hormone levels and perhaps trying some of the alternative, non-hormonal therapies to help reduce your level of symptoms.

If you answered "yes" to four to six questions, you are likely transitioning into the perimenopause, and may be a candidate to begin hormone replacement therapy. See your gynecologist or other health-care provider for help determining your hormone levels to see whether replacement therapy is necessary and to what degree. Consider bone density testing.

If you answered "yes" to seven or more questions, you are almost definitely experiencing significant symptoms of the menopause. You may be at risk for several serious health problems, and should consider hormone replacement therapy as a primary medical treatment, after your risks and benefits are assessed. Bone-density tests should be done and a cardiovascular profile should be taken.

If you answered "yes" to 10 or more questions, walk (don't run, you might injure yourself) to your gynecologist or other health-care provider immediately to request a health checkup, with emphasis on hormone assessment. Chances are, you are well into menopause, and have been for some time. You may already have demonstrated the consequences of hormone deficiency and are at risk for other health problems. All assessments should be done and you should work with your health-care provider to create a health-management plan.

Of course, some of the questions indicate more significant problems than others, but they are all important. Remember, finding the appropriate health-care professional is critical to completing an appropriate evaluation and achieving successful therapy. This quiz will help you identify whether the menopause is a problem for you yet. You can identify the risk factors you possess and options you have for therapy.

APPENDIX F

RESOURCES
Organizations, Books, and Pamphlets

● ● ●

Note: Resources listed here do not imply endorsement by the authors, nor agreement with advice, information or philosophy, or the resource organization.

The North American Menopause Society (NAMS)
P. O. Box 94527
Cleveland, OH 44101
216-844-8748
800-774-5342
http://www.menopause.org/

American Cancer Society
800-ACS-2345 (800-227-2345)
http://www.cancer.org/

American College of Obstetricians and Gynecologists (ACOG)
Resource Center
P. O. Box 96920
Washington, DC 20090-6920
http://www.acog.org/

American Medical Association
Private Sector Hotline: 800-262-3211
Private Sector Fax Line: 312-464-5846
http://www.ama-assn.org/

American Society for Reproductive Health Professionals (ASRM)
209 Montgomery Highway
Birmingham, AL 35216
205-978-5000
http://www.asrm.com/

Association of Women's Health, Obstetric and Neonatal Nurses
(AWHONN)
2000 L Street, NW, Suite 740
Washington, DC 20036
202-261-2400
800-673-8499
http://www.awhonn.org/

Fem-Health, A Perimenopausal Education Resource
EMBRYON
Post Office Plaza
50 Division Street, Suite 501
Somerville, NJ 08876
908-575-1020
http://www.peri-menopause.com/

Menopause Online
http://www.menopause-online.com/

National Association for Professionals in Women's Health (NAPWH)
175 West Jackson Boulevard, A1711
Chicago, IL 60604
312-786-1468
http://www.napwh.org/

National Institutes of Health
Bethesda, MD 20892
301-496-4000
http://www.nih.gov/

National Institutes of Health: National Center for Complementary
and Alternative Medicine
http://nccam.nih.gov/

National Institutes of Health: Office of Dietary Supplements
http://dietary-supplements.info.nih.gov/

National Women's Health Network
514 10th Street, NW, Suite 400
Washington, DC 20004
202-628-7814

National Women's Health Resource Center
http://www.healthywomen.org/

New York Online Access to Health, City University of New York;
New York Public Library, New York Academy of Medicine
http://noah.cuny.edu/

The Society of Obstetricians and Gynecologists of Canada (SOGC)
774 Echo Drive
Ottawa, ON K1S 5N8, Canada
613-730-4192
http://www.medical.org/

The following booklets, books and newsletter were excerpted from the suggested reading list of the North American Menopause Society. For more information and additional reading, visit the NAMS Web site at http://www.menopause.org/ or contact the organization at the address shown below.

BOOKLETS

Menopause Guidebook, 1999. 50 pages. $8.

Induced Menopause Guidebook, 1999. 28 pages. $8.

Menopause: A New Beginning 1998. 26 pages. $8.00.
Available from: The North American Menopause Society
P.O. Box 94527
Cleveland, OH 44101-4527
Toll-free in U.S. and Canada: 800-774-5342
Outside U.S. and Canada: 440-442-7550

Boning Up on Osteoporosis: A Guide to Prevention and Treatment, 1998. 70 pages. $3.
Available from: National Osteoporosis Foundation
P.O. Box 930299
Atlanta, GA 31193-0299
Toll-free in U.S.: 877-868-4520
Outside U.S.: 202-223-2226 (Washington, DC, office)

Managing Menopause: Ways to Relieve Symptoms and Prevent Disease at Midlife, 43 pages. $16.
Available from: Harvard Health Publications
Department SR
P.O. Box 380
Boston, MA 02117

Menopause: Let's Talk About It (1999 ed.); *Osteoporosis: Let's Talk About It* (2000 ed.); *Heart Disease: Let's Talk About It.*
Free.
Available from: The Osteoporosis Society of Canada
33 Laird Drive
Toronto, ON M4G 3S9, Canada
Toll-free in Canada: 800-463-6842 (English); 800-977-1778 (French)
Outside Canada: 416-696-2663

Menopause Handbook, 1997. 50 pages. $5.
Available from: Montreal Health Press Inc.
P.O. Box 1000
Station Place du Parc
Montreal, PQ H2W 2N1, Canada
514-282-1171

Taking Hormones & Women's Health: Choices, Risks and Benefits, 2000. 135 pages. $10/Women's Health Network members. $15/non-members.
Available from: National Women's Health Network
514 10th Street, NW, Suite 400
Washington, DC 20004
202-347-1140

Women & Sleep, 1998. 16 pages. Free w/SASE.
Available from: National Sleep Foundation
1522 K Street, NW, Ste. 500
Washington, DC 20005
Toll-free in U.S.: 888-NSF-SLEEP
Outside U.S.: 202-347-3471

BOOKS

Break the Stress Cycle! 10 Steps to Reducing Stress for Women by Judith Sachs. Holbrook, MA: Adams Media, 1998

CalciYum! Calcium-Rich, Dairy-Free Vegetarian Recipes by David and Rachelle Bronfman, Toronto, ON: Bromedia, 1998

Could It Be . . . Perimenopause? by Steven R. Goldstein, MD, and Laurie Ashner. New York, NY: Little Brown, 1998

Estrogen by Lila E. Nachtigall, MD, and Joan Rattner Heilman. New York, NY: HarperCollins Publishers, 2000 (3rd ed.)

The Healthy Boomer: A No-Nonsense Midlife Guide for Women and Men by Peggy Edwards, Miroslava Lhotsky, MD, and Judy Turner, PhD. Toronto, ON: McClelland & Steward, 1999

I Love Menopause Because . . . by Joyce Silverman Ben-Kiki and Robin Sherman Herman Kansas City, MO: McMeel Publishing, 1998

Menopause and Culture by Gabriella E. Berger. London, England: Pluto Press, 1999

Menopause, Me and You: The Sound of Women Pausing by Ann M. Voda, RN, PhD. Binghampton, NY: Haworth Press, 1997

150 Most-Asked Questions About Menopause: What Women Really Want to Know by Ruth S. Jacobowitz. New York, NY: Morrow, 1996

On Women Turning 50: Celebrating Mid-Life Discoveries by Cathleen Rountree. New York, NY: Harper, 1993

The Osteoporosis Handbook by Sidney Lou Bonnick, MD, FACP Dallas, TX: Taylor, 1997

Our Bodies, Ourselves for the New Century by The Boston Women's Health Book Collective. New York, NY: Touchstone, 1998

The Pause: Positive Approaches to Menopause by Lonnie Barbach, PhD. New York, NY: The Penguin Group, 2000 (rev. ed.)

Perimenopause: Preparing for the Change by Nancy Lee Teaff MD, and Kim Wright Wiley. Rocklin, CA: Prima Publishing, 1999 (2nd ed.)

The Premature Menopause Book: When the "Change of Life" Comes Too Early by Kathryn Petras. New York, NY: Avon Books, 1999 (also has Website at www.prematuremenopause.com)

Stand Tall: Every Woman's Guide to Preventing and Treating Osteoporosis by Morris Notelovitz, MD, PhD, with Marsha Ware, MD, and Diana Tonnessen. (Physical Therapy Consultant: Sara Meeks, PT, GCS) Gainesville, FL: Triad Publishing, 1998 (2nd ed.)

Strong Women Strong Bones by Miriam E. Nelson, PhD, and Sarah Wernick, PhD. New York, NY: G.P. Putnam's Sons, 2000

Successful Aging by John W. Rowe, MD, and Robert L. Kahn, PhD. New York, NY: Dell, 1998

Tell Me What to Eat as I Approach Menopause by Elaine Magee, MPH, RD. Franklin Lakes, NJ: Career Press, 1999

Transformation through Menopause by Marian Van Eyk McCain. New York, NY: Bergin & Garvey, 1991

The Urinary Incontinence Sourcebook by Diane Kaschak Newman, RNC, CRNP, FAAN, with Mary K. Dzurinko. Los Angeles, CA: Lowell House, 1997

Women's Moods: What Every Woman Must Know about Hormones, the Brain, and Emotional Health by Deborah Sichel, MD, and Jeanne Driscoll, MS, RN, CS. New York, NY: William Morrow & Co., Inc., 1999

NEWSLETTERS

Harvard Women's Health Watch
P.O. Box 420068
Palm Coast, FL 32142-0068
Toll-free in U.S.: 800-829-5921;
Outside U.S.: 904-445-4662

GLOSSARY

• • •

NUMBERS

17-beta estradiol   The form of estrogen found naturally in the body.

A

adenomyosis   A condition when defects in the wall of the uterus are found in the muscle, causing abnormal bleeding. *See also endometriosis.*

AIDS   *See HIV/AIDS.*

alendronate   Brand name Fosamax®. A medicine that promotes the development and maintenance of normal bone tissue. A type of bisphosphonate.

Alzheimer's disease   A chronic, progressive form of dementia (loss of mental faculties).

ampicillin   An antibiotic taken for various infections.

androgen   A "male" hormone; for example, testosterone.

androgenic

Literally, "malelike." The usually unwanted appearance of masculine features in a woman, such as a deep voice, facial hair, etc.

androstenedione

A type of androgen.

anemia

Low red blood cell count, usually caused by iron deficiency.

anovulation

Literally, "lack of ovulation." When a woman stops releasing eggs during her monthly cycle.

antidepressant

A medication that boosts mood.

antioxidant

A substance said to prevent oxidation of cells in the tissues, which is a risk for cancer change.

applicator

A device that premeasures medication, such as creams, primarily for vaginal use.

B

bacterial culture

A medium that grows a single bacterium into a large number, so they can be identified.

bacterial vaginosis

A bacterial vaginal infection that causes a gray discharge and "fishy" odor. It is diagnosed by viewing a wet mount of the discharge under a microscope, or by measuring the pH (acidity/alkalinity) of the vagina. It may be treated with metronidazole or ampicillin.

barrier methods

Forms of birth control in which a barrier prevents the sperm from either passing the

collagen

A vital protein in your body that keeps your skin and tissues supple, elastic, and full.

colonoscopy

An examination in which the entire colon is studied through a viewing device inserted through the rectum. This procedure examines more of the colon than a sigmoidoscopy.

colorectal cancer

Cancer of the colon or rectum.

compounding pharmacy

A pharmacy that can prepare custom hormone formulas.

condyloma (venereal warts)

This virus often appears as itchy or painful external warts. It also can appear as a viral injury of the genital tissues and show up as an abnormal Pap smear. It can be spread by an unknowning partner, which results in varying intervals before the time of acquiring the virus and demonstrating any sign of it. It may lie dormant for years, and may result in increased risk of certain genital cancers, including cancer of the cervix. It is usually diagnosed by visual inspection or biopsy and treated by medications or removal (through burning, freezing, or surgical removal).

continuous regimen therapy

Refers to taking drugs on a daily basis, as opposed to "cyclic replacement therapy."

cyclic replacement therapy

Intermittent treatment with predetermined doses for each of several medications, as opposed to "continuous regimen therapy."

D

D&C — Dilation and curettage. Surgical removal of the lining of the uterus.

dementia — A loss of mental function that may be characterized by delusions, drastic loss of memory, and lack of coherency. Usually associated with old age, degenerative neural disease, severe head trauma, and the wrong combination of medications, especially in older women.

Depo-Provera — A type of birth-control medication, taken by a long-acting injection. It provides contraception for up to three months. It may cause irregular bleeding and depression in some women.

designer estrogen — An estrogen product that has been developed to selectively stimulate tissues, thus avoiding bad side effects.

DEXA — Dual-energy x-ray absorptiometry. A method of screening for osteoporosis.

DHEA — Dehydroepiandosterone. A naturally occurring precursor to some of the male hormones, claimed to deliver health benefits. Its risks and benefits are controversial and not yet fully proven. The long-term effects are uncertain.

diabetes — A disease characterized by the body's inability to process sugar in the diet. *Type 1 diabetes* is hereditary, and requires insulin injections to maintain health. *Type 2 diabetes* can sometimes be treated by weight loss, diet, exercise, and oral medication. Sometimes, it too requires insulin. Type 2 diabetes is more likely if you are over 45 years old, have a positive family history, are 20 percent or more over your target body weight, if you are inactive, test low for high-density lipoproteins (HDL, or "good" cholesterol), high for triglycerides, or high for blood pressure.

differentiation

With regard to tumors, the degree of difference between the tumor and the surrounding tissue. Undifferentiated tumors resemble the surrounding tissue; differentiated tumors do not.

dyspareunia

Pain or discomfort during sexual activity.

E

elasticity

Flexibility, "stretchiness," or pliability. In relation to skin or the body, the ability of tissue to stretch easily without discomfort.

endometrial sampling

The removal of cells from the lining of the uterus with a special catheter, to rule out abnormal changes.

endometriosis

When portions of the linings of the uterus implant in the abdomen. Ovaries are the main site of this condition, which may cause internal abnormal bleeding, cyclic with the period. This may result in scar tissue, tubal damage, and pain.

erythromycin

An antibiotic taken for various infections.

estradiol

One of the three main estrogens (E2). Plays a role in tests commonly done to determine a woman's hormone level as it relates to menopause. *See also follicle stimulating hormone.*

Estring®   An estrogen therapy comprised of a flexible
                         ring that is placed in the vagina and releases
                         small amounts of estrogen over three months.

estriol   One of the three main estrogens (E3).
                         Estriol is the weakest of the three main es-
                         trogens and is thought to be less of a cancer
                         risk for breast tissue.

estrogen   A "female" hormone that is produced by
                         multiple organs in a woman's body, but pri-
                         marily by the ovary.

estrogen cream   A formula of estrogen dispersed in various
                         cream bases for topical or vaginal applica-
                         tions.

estrone   One of the three estrogens (E1). Estrone is
                         found in some mixed and plain medica-
                         tions.

Evista®   *See raloxifene.*

F
FDA   Food and Drug Administration. The U.S.
                         federal regulatory agency responsible for
                         setting and measuring safety standards for
                         food and drugs, and for approving drugs
                         for sale.

fibrocystic breast   A common prominence of glands in the
change, fibrocystic   breast, which may result in pain, cyst forma-
disease   tion, and difficulty in examining for cancer
                         screening, because of breast "lumpiness." It
                         is not precancerous.

fibroid   A benign muscle tumor of the uterus.

fish oils	Fish oils contain omega-3 fatty acids. They may act as a blood thinner, and may be used as a potential breast-cancer treatment or preventative. They may lower the risk of colon cancer.
follicle stimulating hormone	One of the hormones commonly tested to determine a woman's hormone level as it relates to menopause. Levels of approximately 20 (depending on the laboratory) are usually diagnostic of menopause. *See also estradiol.*
Fosamax®	*See alendronate.*
frequency	The need to urinate more frequently than normal.
FSH	*See follicle stimulating hormone.*

G

g	g = gram. A metric measurement of weight. About a 28th of an ounce.
GI tract	Gastrointestinal tract. The stomach, and upper and lower intestines.
gonorrhea	A sexually transmitted disease caused by a bacterium and treated with antibiotics. It causes increased risks of fallopian-tube damage, and resulting tubal pregnancies. It appears to increase the risk of contracting HIV. Symptoms range from none, to various vaginal discharges.

H

HDL	High-density lipoproteins; desirable (so-called good) cholesterol.

herbals

A class of botanical substances derived from herb plants, often used for medicinal purposes.

herpes

A sexually transmitted virus that lives in healthy nerve tissue, and forms one or more ulcerlike lesions during an outbreak. Breakouts recur, either frequently or infrequently, usually in the same area, such as the vulva, thigh, or buttocks. Although treatable, it is not curable. Stress can increase breakouts, as can the time just before a period.

HIV/AIDS

Human immunodeficiency virus. The virus that causes AIDS (acquired immune deficiency syndrome). This virus is detected by a blood test. The disease is deadly and can be spread by people who show no symptoms. There may be no outward signs that a person has it for several years. One of the most common early signs of this infection in women is frequent yeast infections. (Of course, getting frequent yeast infections doesn't necessarily mean you are HIV-positive!) The only protection against this disease is the male condom; it is more effective in combination with spermicide.

Hodgkin's disease

A cancer of the lymph nodes.

hormone replacement therapy

Any form of supplemental hormones taken to normalize hormonal balance.

hot flashes (also called "hot flushes" or "power surges")

A feeling of warmth, possibly including sweating, that travels, usually from the chest areas through the neck and into the face, although it may occur anywhere on the body. It is sometimes accompanied by redness and is often triggered by stress, spicy food or heat.

HRT	*See hormone replacement therapy.*
hypertension	Abnormally high blood pressure.
hysterectomy	Surgical removal of the uterus.

I

IU	International Units. Used in measuring doses of many vitamins.
incontinence	Loss of urine or inability to control urination.
insulin	A hormone that controls blood sugar.
intrauterine devices or IUDs	Small devices inserted into the uterus that provide contraception by preventing an egg from implanting in the uterine wall.

K

Kegel exercises	Exercises where pelvic muscles are repeatedly contracted and relaxed, used to tone the muscles that control urine flow. They may also result in improved vaginal sexual function.

L

L	L = liter. A metric measurement of volume. Slightly more than a quart.
LDL	Low-density lipoproteins; undesirable (so-called bad) cholesterol.
libido	Sexual desire.

lipid balance	Having the proper amount of cholesterol—high-density and low-density fats—in the blood.
lipids	Types of fat cells in the blood that include triglycerides and cholesterol.
lymph nodes	Collection of lymph cells located in various parts of the body that filter bacteria, and may be a site for the spread of cancerous cells.

M

mammogram	A low-dose x-ray of the breast that provides early detection of breast-cancer cells.
MAO inhibitor	A type of blood pressure medicine that may conflict with (is contraindicated by) many drugs and supplements.
mcg, mg, mL	mcg = microgram ($1/1,000,000^{th}$ of a gram). mg = milligram, ($1/1000^{th}$ of a gram). mL = milliliter, ($1/1000^{th}$ of a liter). Metric measurements of weight (mcg, mg) and volume (mL).
megadoses	Extremely large doses of a vitamin or other substance, characterized by greatly exceeding the recommended dose or RDA.
menopausal transition	The period of time when female hormone levels start to fall, until they reach a steady state.
menopause	The permanent cessation of menses that occurs after the decline of ovarian function.
migraine	A vascular-type headache, characterized by

unilateral pain, nausea, and vomiting. Often called "sick" headaches.

mixture incontinence
A combination of stress and urge incontinence.

MORE study
Multiple Outcomes of Raloxifene Evaluation. A study intended to provide further evidence of the usefulness of selective estrogen receptor modulators (SERMs), specifically raloxifene, in treating menopause and its related symptoms.

musculoskeletal
Of the muscle and bone systems of the body.

N

natural substances
Substances extracted from plants and animal products that exist in nature.

Nolvadex®
See tamoxifen.

Norplant
A type of birth-control medication that is implanted beneath the skin, and releases hormones for up to five years.

O

ob/gyn
Obstetrician-gynecologist. A doctor who specializes in treatment of the female reproductive system, its related organs, and childbirth, and the diseases and conditions associated with them.

oestrogen
An alternate spelling of estrogen.

optimum pulse
Your ideal rate of heartbeat (pulse) during exercise, calculated with the formula: (220 - your age) x .75

osteopenia — The precursor to osteoporosis. It is a thinning of the bone mass without the actual damage that occurs in osteoporosis.

osteoporosis — Loss of bone severe enough to cause defects in the bone structure, making bones susceptible to fracture.

ovary — The female gonad (reproductive organ), where the egg stores come from.

overflow incontinence — Frequent or constant leakage of urine when the bladder is full.

P

Pap smear — A collection of cervical cells sampled to screen for cancer, hormonal imbalance, and infections.

PapSure® — A new, more accurate Pap test in which the tissue is viewed "live" by the doctor, instead of being sampled, as in a Pap smear.

pelvic ultrasound — Use of sound waves to outline structures in the abdomen, specifically, the uterus and fallopian tubes.

perimenopause — The years surrounding and including menopause.

pessaries — Support devices used to restore the function of organs that have fallen down (prolapsed).

pg — pg = picogram ($1/1,000,000,000,000^{th}$ of a gram). A metric measurement of weight.

Pill, the — *See birth-control pill.*

placebo effect

An effect noticed in medical studies where a placebo (i.e., a sugar pill, or non-active treatment) seems to cure or improve a condition. In effect the condition improves by itself, through mental power.

polyps

Small protrusions of cells from the cervix or uterus that form fingerlike projections that may bleed or require removal.

postpartum blues

A commonly occurring, mild depression that is temporary, occurring briefly after childbirth. It is not life-threatening and resolves spontaneously.

postpartum depression

A serious, possibly life-threatening condition in new mothers, characterized by severe depression following childbirth, thought to be caused by the radical drop in hormones, particularly estrogen. It can be treated by estrogen, but may also require antidepressant therapy.

postpartum psychosis

A more extreme disorder than postpartum depression, postpartum psychosis may be a mania, or may be a bipolar disorder (manic-depression). It requires immediate psychiatric evaluation and treatment.

power surge

A euphemism or alternate phrase for "hot flash." *(See also hot flash.)*

Premarin®

Brand name for a form of estrogen.

premature menopause

In medical terminology, menopause that occurs before age 40, or in reality, anytime before you're ready for it.

premature ovarian failure | When the ovaries stop producing estrogen at a young age. May be due to genetics, disease, or extreme stress, such as surgery.

progesterone | A primarily "female" hormone, responsible for the shedding of the lining of the uterus after estrogen has built it up, creating the period.

progestin | A synthetic hormone similar to progesterone, but not identical.

prolactin | The hormone that causes the production of milklike substances from the breast. It is elevated in pregnancy and some tumors.

prolapse | When an organ loses structural strength, causing it to fall partially out of its place.

Q

QCT | Quantitative computed tomography. A method of screening for osteoporosis.

R

raloxifene (Evista®) | A "designer estrogen" designed to have positive effects on bones and lipids but apparently does not increase stimulation of endometrial or breast tissues.

RDA | Recommended Daily Allowance. The recommended amount of a vitamin, mineral, or other nutrient that you should strive to get each day.

receptor | Locations on the cells of organs in the body where drugs and normal physiological chemicals "bind."

regimen base

The appropriate balance of hormone or treatment dosages that works best for you.

RUTH study

Raloxifene Use for the Heart. A study intended to provide further evidence of the usefulness of selective estrogen receptor modulators (SERMs), specifically raloxifene and its potential cardiovascular benefits

S

salivary hormone tests

A method of measuring hormone levels using fluids taken from the salivary glands of the mouth.

screening chart

A chart for tracking the health of a patient. *See Appendix C.*

SERMS

Selective estrogen receptor modulators. These are substances that selectively affect the estrogen receptors in your body, so, for example, the receptors that increase your bone density are stimulated, but the receptors that stimulate your breast tissue are not.

sex steroid hormone binding globulin (SHBG)

Blood cells that attach or bind themselves to hormones in the bloodstream.

sigmoidoscopy

An examination in which the colon is studied through a viewing device inserted through the rectum. This procedure does not examine as much of the colon as a colonoscopy.

sleep apnea

A condition that causes you to wake up frequently because you repeatedly stop breathing; also contributes to sleep fragmentation.

sleep fragmentation   When your sleep is frequently interrupted during the night.

soy protein   A natural protein, derived from soybeans, commonly used as a supplement to provide natural phytoestrogens.

sterilization   A process that results in a person being unable to conceive children. It may be surgical, disease-related, or naturally occurring. Surgical sterilization is considered a radical, usually permanent method of birth control.

STD   Sexually transmitted disease. A disease spread through sexual contact.

St. John's wort   A natural herbal product used for mood elevation (as an antidepressant).

stress incontinence   Leakage of urine caused by activity, shaking, coughing, etc. It may be triggered simply by lifting something, or even by the stepping action of climbing stairs.

subdermal   Under the skin. Subdermal therapies (such as Norplant) allow medications to be implanted under the skin and released slowly over time.

surgical menopause   A premature menopause caused by the sudden drop in estrogen production that may occur when: (a) one or both ovaries are removed, and/or (b) the uterus is removed.

synthetic substances   Substances that are chemically derived without a natural source.

syphilis   A sexually transmitted disease diagnosed by

a blood test called VDRL and treated with antibiotics. If left untreated, it can lead to serious neurological problems and death. The main symptom is usually a large, painless ulcer on the genitals.

T

tamoxifen (Nolvadex®)

A chemotherapy treatment for breast cancer, and in breast-cancer prevention trials, that appears to have an antiestrogen effect on breast tissue, and an estrogen-like effect on bones. It may increase risk of uterine cancer.

testosterone

A primarily "male" hormone or *androgen*, produced in small amounts by several organs of the female body as well, including the ovaries.

tetracycline

An antibiotic taken for various infections.

thromboembolisms

Blood clots in the lung or legs.

thrombophlebitis

Inflammation of certain blood vessels, accompanied by pain and swelling.

thyroid hormone

A hormone produced by the thyroid gland that, among other things, is responsible for the rate of metabolism.

titrate, titration

To adjust medication in increments to adapt to the individual result required.

transdermal

Through the skin. Transdermal therapies, such as patches, allow medication to be absorbed directly through the skin.

trichomoniasis

A parasitic infection diagnosed by taking a

small sample of vaginal discharge and ob-serving it through a microscope on what is called a "wet mount." It is treated with metronidazole. Trichomoniasis can increase the risk of HIV and causes little red dots on the cervix and vagina.

triestrogen

Blends of three types of estrogen, such as 10 percent estrone, 10 percent estradiol, and 80 percent estriol. *(See also biestrogen.)*

triglycerides

Fats in the blood. Thought to be improved by estrogen therapy.

T-score

A measure of absolute bone mass, used to measure osteoporosis, based on bone mass relative to young adult mean.
–1.0 and above = young, normal bones
–1.0 and –2.5 = osteopenia
–2.5 or less = possible osteoporosis

tubal ligation (Band-Aid sterilization)

Also known as "having your tubes tied." A form of sterilization where the fallopian tubes are interrupted, using a technique per-formed through very small abdominal inci-sions.

tumor grade

A description of severity of cell type in a cancer.

U

ultrasonography

The technical term for ultrasound.

ultrasound

Any use of sound waves to image parts of the body.

urethra

A part of the urinary tract; the tube leading from the bladder to the outside of the body.

urge incontinence	A frequent strong feeling you need to urinate right away, sometimes accompanied by loss of urine.
urgency	The need to urinate more urgently. *See also urge incontinence.*
urinary incontinence	*See incontinence.*
urinary tract	The kidneys, ureters, urethra, and bladder.
urinary-tract infection	An overgrowth of bacteria in the bladder or anywhere in the urinary tract.
uterus	In women, the main reproductive organ where fertilized eggs implant and develop. The womb.

V

vagina	Part of the female reproductive system; specifically, the passage from the vulva to the cervix.
vasomotor symptoms	*See hot flashes.*
virilization	An unwanted side effect of male hormones, such as acne, oily skin, deepening of voice, or hair growth.
vitamin E	A vitamin thought to be an antioxidant. Thought to be useful in decreasing fibrocystic breast pain and hot flashes.
vulva	The external (visible) female sex organs.
vulvar	Of, or relating to, the vulva.

W

wet mount | A type of preparation on a glass slide used in the evaluation of a substance under a microscope. Typically, a preparation of normal saline solutions and bodily fluids (e.g., vaginal secretions or discharges) viewed under a microscope. Often used to examine bodily fluids for bacteria.

WHI | Women's Health Initiative. A study to provide further evidence of the usefulness of selective estrogen receptor modulators (SERMs) in treating menopause and its related symptoms by examining estrogen and hormone replacement therapy in general.

WISDOM | Women's International Study of Long Duration Oestrogen (estrogen) after Menopause. It will examine estrogen and hormone replacement therapy in general.

withdrawal bleeding | Bleeding from the uterus that occurs as the result of a significant drop in hormone levels.

Y

yeast infections | Benign fungal infections usually treated with creams or pills. Commonly noticed first as a red, bumpy, itchy rash around the genitals, on the thighs, or even under the breasts. Yeast infections may be diagnosed by analysis of a vaginal discharge under a microscope.

Z

Z-score | A measure of bone mass, used to diagnose and measure the degree of osteoporosis.

NOTES

• • •

[1] "Bisphosphonates for treating and preventing osteoporosis." Salvatori, Roberto and Levine, Michael A, *Contemporary OB/GYN*. April 1998.

[2] "Bisphosphonates for treating and preventing osteoporosis." Salvatori, Roberto and Levine, Michael A, *Contemporary OB/GYN*. April 1998.

[3] "Bisphosphonates for treating and preventing osteoporosis." Salvatori, Roberto and Levine, Michael A, *Contemporary OB/GYN*. April 1998.

[4] "Women of Color at Risk for Low Bone Mass and Osteoporosis," *NAPWH FOCUS*, Vol. II, No. 3, Winter 1999.

[5] "Bisphosphonates for treating and preventing osteoporosis." Salvatori, Roberto and Levine, Michael A, *Contemporary OB/GYN*. April 1998.

[6] "Prevention and Treatment of Postmenopausal Osteoporosis." *PCS RxReview*. December 1997.

[7] "Cardiovascular Disease in Women." *Clinical Courier*, Vol. 16, No. 32, February 1998.

[8] Menopause Guidebook, *Helping You Make Informed Healthcare Decisions at Midlife*, North American Menopause Society (1998).

[9] Menopause Guidebook, *Helping You Make Informed Healthcare Decisions at Midlife*, North American Menopause Society (1998).

[10] *TMB (The Menopause Book?)*, p158.

[11] PCS Health Systems, *PCS RxReview*, "Prevention and Treatment of Postmenopausal Osteoporosis." Quoting the following three sources: (1) "Conference Report, Consensus Development Conference: Diagnosis, prophylaxis, and treatment of osteoporosis." *Am J Med*. 1993; 94:646–50. (2) Ray NF, Chan JK, Thamer M, Melton LJ. "Medical expenditures for the treatment of osteoporotic fractures in the United States in 1995: Report from the National Osteoporosis Foundation." *J Bone Miner Res*. 1997; 12:24–35. (3) Samsioe G. "Osteoporosis–an update." *Acta Obstet Gynecol Scand*. 1997; 76:189–199.

[12] PCS Health Systems, *PCS RxReview*, "Prevention and Treatment of Postmenopausal Osteoporosis." Quoting the following source: Riggs BL, Melton LJ. "The prevention and treatment of osteoporosis." *N Engl J Med*. 1992; 327(9); 620–627.

[13] "Seven steps to the effective treatment of osteoporosis in your practice," Barbieri, Robert L., MD. *Contemporary OB/GYN*. February 1998.

[14] "Bisphosphonates and Osteoporosis," *Contemporary OB/Gyn,* April 1998. Quoting Melton LJ III, Chrischilles EA, Cooper C, et al. "How many women have osteoporosis?" *J Bone Miner Res.* 1992; 7:1005–1010.

[15] "Women of Color at Risk for Low Bone Mass and Osteoporosis," *NAPWH FOCUS,* Vol. 11, No. 3, Winter 1999.

[16] "Preventing Falls in Elderly Women," Research Report, WOMEN'S HEALTH in *Primary Care,* June, 1999. Vol. 2, No. 6.

[17] "Mood, Cognition, and Dementia: Effects of Postmenopausal Hormone Therapy," *Contemporary Ob/Gyn,* February 1998.

[18] "Mood, Cognition, and Dementia: Effects of Postmenopausal Hormone Therapy," *Contemporary Ob/Gyn,* February 1998.

[19] Alzheimer's Disease in Women," Annlia Paganini-Hill, Ph.D., *The Female Patient®,* Vol. 23, March 1998, quoting Hampson E. "Variations in sex related cognitive abilities across the menstrual cycle." *Brain Cogn.* 1990; 14:26–43; Phillips SM, Sherwin BB. "Variations in memory and sex steroid hormones across the menstrual cycle." *Psychoneuroendocrinology.* 1992; 17:497–506; and Krug R, Stamm U, Pietrowsky R, et al. "Effects of menstrual cycle on creativity. *Psychoneuroendocrinology.* 1994; 19:21–31.

[20] Alzheimer's Disease in Women," Annlia Paganini-Hill, Ph.D., *The Female Patient®,* Vol. 23, March 1998.

[21] *Menopause Guidebook, Helping You Make Informed Healthcare Decisions at Midlife,* North American Menopause Society (1998).

[22] "Vitamins and Multivitamins—What Are the Benefits?" Greenwood, Sadja, MD MPH, *Menopause Management,* March/April 1999.

[23] *Ob. Gyn. News,* November 1, 1998—"Foods Serve as Adjuncts to HRT;" Johnson, Kate.

[24] "Women's Health . . . in the news." July 19, 1999. [citing *Cancer Epidemiology, Biomarkers and Prevention,* July 1999.]

[25] Ibid.

[26] *Ob. Gyn. News,* November 1, 1998.

[27] *Menopause Guidebook, Helping You Make Informed Healthcare Decisions at Midlife,* North American Menopause Society (1998).

Index